UNDERSTANDING HEALING

MEDITATIVE REFLECTIONS ON DEEPENING
MEDICINE THROUGH SPIRITUAL SCIENCE

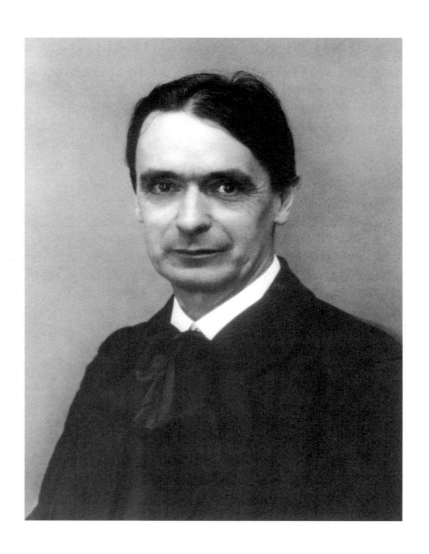

UNDERSTANDING HEALING

MEDITATIVE REFLECTIONS ON DEEPENING MEDICINE THROUGH SPIRITUAL SCIENCE

Thirteen lectures and a meeting held in Dornach between January and
April 1924
First Newsletter of the Medical Section, March 1924

TRANSLATED BY CHRISTIAN VON ARNIM

INTRODUCTION BY CHRISTIAN VON ARNIM

RUDOLF STEINER

RUDOLF STEINER PRESS

CW 316

The publishers acknowledge the generous funding of this publication by Dr Eva Frommer MD (1927–2004) and the Anthroposophical Society in Great Britain

Rudolf Steiner Press
Hillside House, The Square
Forest Row, RH18 5ES

www.rudolfsteinerpress.com

Published by Rudolf Steiner Press 2013

Originally published in German under the title *Meditative Betrachtungen und Anleitungen zur Vertiefung der Heilkunst* (volume 316 in the *Rudolf Steiner Gesamtausgabe* or Collected Works) by Rudolf Steiner Verlag, Dornach. Based on notes taken by members of the audiences not reviewed by the speaker, and edited by Hans W. Zbinden, MD. This authorized translation is based on the 5th German edition of 2008 which was overseen by Andreas Dollfuss and Eva-Gabriele Streit, MD

Published by permission of the Rudolf Steiner Nachlassverwaltung, Dornach

© Rudolf Steiner Nachlassverwaltung, Dornach 1967, Rudolf Steiner Verlag 2008

This translation © Rudolf Steiner Press 2013

A catalogue record for this book is available from the British Library

ISBN 978 1 85584 381 3

Cover by Mary Giddens
Typeset by DP Photosetting, Neath, West Glamorgan
Printed and bound in Great Britain by Gutenberg Press Ltd., Malta

CONTENTS

CHRISTMAS COURSE

LECTURE 1
DORNACH, 2 JANUARY 1924

Illusion of imagining the human being as firmly outlined. The physically outlined human being. The fluid human being on which the etheric body acts; the aeriform human being in which the astral body works; the warmth human being which penetrates the human organization. The I works on the warmth human being whereas the latter acts on the rest of the organization, the I therefore does so indirectly. That provides true insight into the relationship between soul and spirit as the soul events act on the warmth ether and through the latter on the organs.

The possibility of falling ill lies in the human organization. The possibility of healing in natural processes which can take over the processes in the human being: etheric body, astral body, I. Calling on higher components of the human being to aid healing. Natural science has to look at things in a different way to accord with the living-cosmic aspect; example of formic acid and the way that figs ripen and honey is produced. Necessity of developing a feeling for nature, also when using a microscope. Consideration of size which is not relative. A look at the real nature of the beehive.

LECTURE 2
DORNACH, 3 JANUARY 1924

Characterization of the components of the human being. I and earthly form. I and death. Physical organism and nourishment. Relationship between etheric body and astral body and the possibility of falling ill. Prerequisite for a conscious soul life. The nature of feeling. The development of illness. Inflammation and excess growth. Illness and the soul life. Liver as the sense organ for the substances of the external world. Heart, a sense organ for the inner world. The organs as intrinsic whole. Assessment of food from the global context of the human organism.

LECTURE 3
DORNACH, 4 JANUARY 1924

The forces which come from the earth and the forces which come from the periphery are balanced in the individual organ systems. The head from this perspective; its weightlessness and state of static rest. Cosmic and earthly forces in the head and skeleton. The importance of calcium carbonate and calcium phosphate. Substances as cosmic formative forces and the behaviour of the cosmic essence in that regard. Special consideration of the forces which overcome the lead process. The importance of the magnesium process, rhythmical periods in which the process has a different meaning. Antimony and the metamorphoses of the coal process studied in accordance with cosmic and etheric formative processes in time.

LECTURE 4
DORNACH, 5 JANUARY 1924

Exoteric knowledge and the way it is acquired as the basis for the esoteric part of the course. Development of the human being: the etheric body and its relationship with the embryo which is created through heredity, its relationship with the astral body in the period immediately after birth: predisposition for knowledge. Importance of inner schooling and deepening for the physician who wants to heal. Care of the soul forces through rhythmical repetition of knowledge. Such knowledge is illustrated using the example of experiencing a plant, exoteric and esoteric knowledge put into their real context.

LECTURE 5
DORNACH, 6 JANUARY 1924

About the change which has to occur in the whole attitude of the anthroposophical movement: 'The esoteric path is a difficult one or it is none at all.' Further description of the cosmic forces by means of the example of the relationship between the nature of plants and the human organism, particularly the head.

Necessity of experiencing such knowledge. Connecting this with inner moral impulses. Description of meditative processes. The will to deepen medical studies esoterically in the same way as has happened so far only in two areas: general anthroposophy and the arts of eurythmy and speech. Description of the way the Medical Section is set up.

LECTURE 6

DORNACH, 7 JANUARY 1924

Cognition through the thoughts: skeletal system; through imagination: fluid human being, muscular system. Cognition through intuition: warmth human being and the activity of the organs. The two types of warmth. Aerifom and light state. Metamorphosis of light. Water and the chemical metabolism. The earthy and life. Conceptual medical knowledge and the therapeutic element.

LECTURE 7

DORNACH, 8 JANUARY 1924

Answer to a question about magnetic healing. Answer to a question about the relationship between the heart and uterus. Answer to a question about the influence of precious stones on the individual organs. Answer to a question about the effect of post-mortem decomposition processes on the deceased. Answer to a question about the effect of a post-mortem examination for a certain period after death. Answer to a question of the importance of community for the healing abilities of physicians. Answer to a question about iris diagnosis, graphology and so on. About healing and a knowledge of medicines. About the nature of the book *Philosophy of Freedom* and its meaning with regard to the nature of the human being. Imagination and the muscles; inspiration and the life of the inner organs. Outline of the course of study deemed necessary by Rudolf Steiner for a medicine which accords with the spirit. The nature of illness for the physician with the will to heal.

LECTURE 8

DORNACH, 9 JANUARY 1924

Karma as a guide for the physician: the will that karma be fulfilled and the will to heal. Introduction to the way of viewing the human organism leading to healing as the result of cosmic forces, illustrated using the example of Saturn and moon forces. Instructions for meditative deepening.

Pages 97–112

EASTER COURSE

LECTURE 9

DORNACH, 21 APRIL 1924

Participants are encouraged to ask questions about difficulties which have arisen when the physician was following an esoteric path of schooling. Answers. Emancipation of the western esoteric path from the external cosmos. Instruction for meditation; about the nature of the latter. Explanation of the incarnation process, development of a human body suitable for earth; origin of the hereditary stream and examination of the latter. The nature of scarlet fever and measles; importance of the child's food and breast milk. Importance of direct perception with regard to meditative knowledge; explanation of the same with examples. Obtaining maturity on earth. The seven-year periods as new elements. The influence of the cosmic formative forces. Meditation on the nature of the plant.

Pages 113–129

LECTURE 10

DORNACH, 22 APRIL 1924

About meditating in the right way and the medical profession. Illness as an aspect of understanding healing. Knowledge about healing and the will to heal. Understanding the etheric as something sculptural. Understanding the astral as something musical. The pioneering role in a new medical course of physicians with an anthroposophical orientation. Observation of the primary cause of disease in the patient biography. Meditation.

Pages 130–144

LECTURE 11

DORNACH, 23 APRIL 1924

Introduction to the meditation given in Lecture 10: the creation of form, the creation of the human being from out of cosmic forces. Moon. Ensouling the human being: the action of the sun out of the cosmos in the environment. The human being filled with spirit through the catabolic forces of Saturn action. The cosmic nature of the forces of the metals. Morality as a force streaming in from the cosmos. Spiritual truths must be repeatedly experienced meditatively. On the karmic situation of the souls born around the turn of the century which seek the spirit.

LECTURE 12
DORNACH, 24 APRIL 1924

The origins of the nineteenth and twentieth century medical point of view looked at in their karmic connections. Christianity and Arabism. Instructions for a healer meditation: the cosmic trinity of Saturn, sun and moon at work in the healthy and sick human being.

Instructions for becoming aware of the karmic situation in patients: the will to heal, imbuing medicine with Christianity by becoming aware of the cosmic aspect in the human being. Involvement of the heart in the thinking: the staff of Mercury. The physician should work towards karma being able to come to expression in contemporary culture.

LECTURE 13
DORNACH, 25 APRIL 1924

The nature of the components of the human being and their reciprocal relation-ships. General causes of falling ill, understanding the action of certain medicines. Different circumstances in physical and mental disease, the temperaments.

Instruction for a meditation to acquire imaginative consciousness. The same for the acquisition of inspirational consciousness. Feeling in knowledge, feeling in cognition. Giving the youth movement a more concrete form through help in the spirit of a medicine striving as described previously. The unobtrusive healing of the hereditary forces in education. Relationship of the physician with the patient. Appeal for an inner connection with the Goetheanum which has set itself a certain task as the centre.

FIRST NEWSLETTER
11 MARCH 1924

Published by the Medical Section of the School of Spiritual Science at the Goetheanum for the anthroposophical physicians and medical students.

EVENING MEETING

DORNACH, 24 APRIL 1924

Relationship between the fluid and solid in the development of the organic. Image creation through extension (cosmic effect) and invagination (earthly effect). The therapeutically important phantom of the organs in the fluid human being. Sculptural principle for understanding the fluid, musical principle for understanding the aeriform. Listening to one another when speaking: study of the I-organization.

Page 195

EDITOR'S PREFACE

At the initiative of a number of physicians who had heard Rudolf Steiner's public lecture 'Die geistewissenschaftliche Grundlage der leiblichen und seelischen Gesundheit' ('The spiritual scientific foundations of physical and mental health', in GA 334, *Social Issues*) in Basel on 6 January 1920, Rudolf Steiner gave a first course on medical subjects in the spring of the same year (see GA 312, *Introducing Anthroposophical Medicine*). A second course followed one year later (GA 313, *Illness and Therapy*) and in parallel a course on eurythmy therapy (GA 315, *Eurythmy Therapy*) which was attended by physicians and eurythmists. After a 'Medical Week' organized by the Clinical and Therapeutic Institute in Stuttgart in October 1922, a small group of younger physicians approached Rudolf Steiner with the request to give a course for the 'young ones' which should be 'quite intimate and not [contain anything] which appealed only to knowledge and the intellect' (Norbert Glas). As a result, the so-called 'young physicians course' was held at the start of 1924 and continued at Easter. These two courses form the content of the present volume. Also included is an address which Rudolf Steiner gave at the evening meeting of the course participants on 24 April 1924, the newsletter from the Medical Section which was sent to participants after the Christmas course, as well as the meditation for physicians mentioned therein.

The chronological table of medical lectures and discussions (over) offers an overview of Rudolf Steiner's lecturing activities in this field:

[GA = Collected works in German]

Date	Venue	Occasion
21 March–9 April 1920	Dornach	First medical course (*Introducing Anthroposophical Medicine*) GA 312
26 March 1920 7 April 1920	Dornach	Q&A on Psychiatry Hygiene as a social issue (both GA 314, *Physiology and Healing*)
7–9 October 1920	Dornach	Lectures on 'Physiological and therapeutic themes based on spiritual science' (GA 314)
11–18 April 1921	Dornach	Second medical course, GA 313 (*Illness and Therapy*)
12–18 April 1921	Dornach	Eurythmy therapy lectures for physicians and eurythmists, GA 315 (*Eurythmy Therapy*)
26–28 October 1922 28 October 1922	Stuttgart	Anthroposophical Basis for the Practice of Medicine (GA 314) Lecture on eurythmy therapy (GA 314)
31 December 1923/ 1 January/2 January 1924	Dornach	Discussions with anthroposophical physicians on Therapy (GA 314)
28 August 1923–29 August 1924	(various cities)	*The Healing Process* (GA 319)
2–9 January 1924	Dornach	GA 316 (*Understanding Healing*)
21–25 April 1924 21–23 April 1924	Dornach	Easter course, part of above (GA 316) Discussions with medical practitioners (GA 314)
25 June–7 July 1924	Dornach	GA 317 (*Education for Special Needs*)
8–18 September 1924	Dornach	GA 318 (*Broken Vessels*)

Summary of Medical Courses in English Translation (latest editions shown):

GA/CW 312   *Introducing Anthroposophical Medicine* (SteinerBooks 2010)

313   *Illness and Therapy* (Rudolf Steiner Press 2013)

314   *Physiology and Healing* (Rudolf Steiner Press 2013)

315   *Eurythmy Therapy* (Rudolf Steiner Press 2009)

316   *Understanding Healing* (Rudolf Steiner Press 2013)

317   *Education for Special Needs* (Rudolf Steiner Press 1998)

318   *Broken Vessels* (SteinerBooks 2003)

319   *The Healing Process* (SteinerBooks 2000)

INTRODUCTION

Of all the fields in which Rudolf Steiner was active—and there were many of them—medicine is probably one of the areas in which it is hardest for the modern scientific mind to accept the basis on which anthroposophy, and Steiner's systematic research into the spirit through spiritual science, operates. As conventional medicine becomes ever more highly technologized—in one development doctors are diagnosing patients remotely via a robot, literally losing touch with them—it sees the human being physically and mentally as no more than the sum of his or her cellular and neuronal parts and processes.

It requires a fundamental shift of paradigm to see human beings, in sickness and health, embedded not just in an earthly but also a spiritual-cosmic setting. Yet that is the starting point for anthroposophic medicine, both in terms of its understanding of the structure of human beings themselves, and of the influences acting on them and the earth from out of the cosmos as planetary forces. Steiner explained the human being very specifically as consisting not just of a physical body but also of what he called the etheric body or life forces, the astral body providing sentience and consciousness, and the I-organization the self-aware, eternal spiritual part of the human being.

This also gives a different perspective on illness and disease. Rather than just being a malfunction of an organ or body part, illness can also be understood as a dislocation of the action of the various components in the human being. In such a case healing in turn involves restoring such activity to its rightful sphere. An organic illness is thus a symptom of such an underlying imbalance, an absence of the harmonious interaction of the human components in the affected organ or organ system. In this view, the physician has to have an understanding of the way in which etheric body, astral body and I-organization positively and negatively impact on one another. In order to make a full diagnosis, the physician has to look beyond just the physical body and have a sharp eye for the human soul life, says Steiner.

But in order to do that, the physician also has to work on himself or herself meditatively, in order to develop the faculties to see beyond the physical person. In these lectures Steiner therefore emphasizes that becoming a physician is not just a profession but a calling. He repeatedly refers to the *will to heal* as a moral quality which the physician needs to develop through meditative work, and discusses the meditations which he gave to help physicians work on their own development.

As a result of these factors, anthroposophic medicine is an individualized medicine. It is not enough to find standard solutions in response to standard diagnoses. The particular constellation of a disease has to be looked at individually in each person, which will also affect the treatment prescribed.

Steiner spends a lot of time in these lectures speaking about the influence of the cosmic and earthly forces, the periphery and the centre, on the human being. These are forces which affect both the human being and the earth itself, so if the physician understands these processes properly, it will also help him or her to understand the actions of the plants and minerals used in anthroposophic and homoeopathic medicines and to choose the appropriate medicine to treat the specific condition of the patient.

In short, in these lectures Steiner paints an extensive picture of the human being as a complex entity formed by forces of heredity from the parents in the physical body (which have to be overcome), forces from the cosmos and by a person's own spiritual individuality, whose task it is to take hold of all the other components and shape them for its own purpose. The physician has to understand these relationships before he or she can start to heal them when they get out of balance.

But what also emerges from these lectures is that Steiner did not see anthroposophic medicine as competing with or wanting to replace conventional medicine. He recognized the achievements of the latter and saw anthroposophic medicine as complementing and extending them—adding the dimension that is absent: namely a non-materialistic and comprehensive view of the human being.

That does not, however, mean that he could not be extremely

scathing about aspects of the medical establishment and what he saw as its stupidities and blinkered attitudes. He was nevertheless quite clear that however unsatisfactory the medical students attending his courses in Dornach found their conventional medical studies, they should undertake and complete them. In an ideal world we might not want to start from where we are—and Steiner does indeed set out how he thinks an ideal medical course should be structured, both in its exoteric and esoteric content.

But he also understood that we are where we are, and therefore have to start from that place. The last thing he wanted was for anthroposophic medicine to be seen as dilettantish and unprofessional, and so he insisted on properly qualified physicians in the way that the world at large demands and recognizes, who would then complement their conventional medical training with the additional insights they gained through the medical courses based on the findings of spiritual science.

So Steiner maintained that while anthroposophical medical students should certainly not be embarrassed to represent the anthroposophical view of the human being—outlandish as it might appear to the conventionally trained scientific mind—it was just as necessary for them to concern themselves with orthodox science and medicine because that, too, was a requirement for healing even if, 'it is the case that in major and significant things the truth diverges considerably from what is accepted today', as Steiner puts it.

Christian von Arnim, July 2013

CHRISTMAS COURSE

LECTURE 1

DORNACH, 2 JANUARY 1924

My dear friends,
The first thing I would like to discuss with you is related to the study of medicine itself. Medical studies today are structured in such a way that they build on a natural scientific view of the world, or rather, a natural scientific interpretation which fails to develop a proper understanding of the human being. And so young physicians see an ill person without being able to develop any real idea about what the healthy human being is like. Because, you see, if you begin by learning about anatomy and physiology with the idea that the key parts of the human organism are the organs and organ systems which appear in firm outline, such as the bone structure and the muscular system, and if you have become used to seeing those systems in the fixed outlines in which they are normally drawn, that gives you a quite erroneous view of the human being. For the things which are drawn in this way and which we imagine as being drawn in this way, what is considered to be the real content of our knowledge, they are engaged in a constant process of development, of generation and degeneration, they are in continuous development, constant coming into being and passing away. And if we now begin to look at this coming into being and passing away, we immediately notice that we have to move away from the fixed outlines in the human organism to something that is fluid and without contours, that we have to imagine the human being as the result of a flow which persists at certain points. And we have to add the fluid human being, if I can put it like that, to that part of the human being which is the least part; we

have to add the human being who is no longer subject to the laws to which sharply outlined bodies are subject.

The opinion is commonly expressed today, on the basis of anatomical and physiological thinking, that when we drink liquid to satisfy our thirst and then drink more and more liquid, say a third or fourth glass after the first one, all the liquid we have drunk undergoes the same process in the organism. But that is not true. The first glass of water undergoes a complicated process to satisfy our thirst; but the second glass of water, when our thirst is no longer so great, passes through the organism at a much greater rate than the first one. It does not follow the complicated progression which the first one did and with the second glass of water we are dealing to a much greater extent with a kind of simple onward flow in the fluid human being, if I can broadly express it like that.

And so we have to say that a true understanding of the human being must, first, take the sharply outlined organs into account, but then also those things which are in flow in the organism. Of course reference is also made to those things which are in flow but it is done in a way which only seeks to understand the fluids, indeed the whole fluid configuration of the human organism, in greater detail on the basis of the laws of dynamics and mechanics. It is not the case that the latter apply; as soon as we consider the fluid human being, the so-called human etheric body is involved.

The human physical body is merely that aspect which relates to the anatomical drawings which you can see in the anatomical dictionaries, the books of anatomy. But you will not find the flow of the fluids in the human organism there. The flow of fluids in the human organism is not dependent on earthly forces—earthly forces are also involved but it is not dependent in its essence on earthly forces—but on those planetary forces which I spoke about in the lecture,[1] so that we have to say: as long as we are dealing with organs and organ systems with a fixed contour, we are only dealing with the earthly forces. [Plate 1* left] As soon as we are dealing with what circulates, be it the circulation of the nutritional fluids themselves or the nutritional fluids that have already

---

* See p. 204 regarding the blackboard drawings.

been transformed into blood, we are dealing with controlling forces that are not earthly but planetary. We will deal with the matter in greater detail later on, but right now we are looking at the principle.

So essentially we have the solid human being associated with the physical body, the fluid human being associated with the etheric body. Now there is also the aeriform, gaseous aspect to the human organism—and to a greater extent than some people think. In so far as the gaseous is in our organism as a constitutional, vitalizing element, it is dependent on the astral body so that, for example, human respiration must be understood in its physical manifestation as a function of the astral body.

And specifically with regard to the fourth human being, the warmth human being—I have referred to the physical human being linked with the physical body, the fluid human being linked with the etheric body, the gaseous human being, i.e. the activity of all that is gaseous or aeriform, linked with the astral body—there cannot be a moment's doubt that in the physical space occupied by the human being, and even beyond, there are different degrees of warmth. If you take someone's temperature behind the ear or in the armpit you will find a very differentiated warmth organism. The degrees of warmth are different everywhere. [Plate 1 right] Just as you can say that the liver is in a specific location in the human being, so you can say that the intestines are in a specific location. Both have quite different temperatures. The liver temperature is quite different as the liver has a very specific warmth organization. This warmth organization is originally linked with the I-organization. Only now, really, is it possible for you to picture the human being to the extent that he or she carries the substances which are otherwise present on earth within himself or herself as solid, fluid, gaseous and warmthlike substances.

The warmth element is directed by the I-organization. But if something is in a particular warmth state, this warmth state has an effect on the thing that is penetrated by the warmth; and this is where we get to the real state of the I-organization. The things which the I-organization otherwise does in the human organism happen by way of the warmth organization. Let us assume that I am walking, just walking. In walking, I act on the warmth organization of my organism with my I-organization. What the warmth does in the organism—in the same way that the legs contain fluids between the solid parts of the legs—is an indirect consequence of the I-organization; but the I-organization only acts directly on the warmth organism. We can therefore see the action of the I-organization in the whole organism—in the solid, fluid, gaseous and warmth organization—but only by way of the warmth organization. We can, in turn, see the action of the astral body on the whole organism, but directly the astral body acts only on our aeriform organization, and so on. You can work out the rest for yourself.

Now you see, this opens up quite a different possibility. Take the kind of thing that is provided in physiology and anatomy today, which people outline so nicely and take to be the whole human being. If you take that you will never have the possibility to get from the human being in this form, who cannot in reality exist, to the soul element or, indeed, the spiritual. How in all the world could anything of a soul or spiritual nature have anything to do with the human being as he or she is outlined today in physiology and anatomy? As a result all kinds of apparently well-considered theories have arisen about the reciprocal relationship between the soul and spirit and the physical. The most ingenious, because the most silly of them—the two things are often connected in our time—is the theory about psychophysical parallelism. It says that both run simultaneously and in parallel and there is no attempt to seek a bridge between them. But as soon as you rise to organized warmth differentiation, and have the intervention of the I-organization in such warmth differentiation, you will realize that it is quite feasible that the I-organization acts on the warmth ether; and that it acts on the whole human being as far down as the sharply contoured physical organization by way of the warmth organization. The only reason that the bridge between the physical and the soul elements in the human being cannot be found is that people ignore that the human being has this consecutive structure which in turn is acted on by the soul and spiritual organization. It is indeed the case that if you experience fear, for example, such a simple mental state initially has an effect on your warmth organization. You cannot of course conceive that the mental fact of experiencing fear makes your limbs shake, that is inconceivable, and so you have to look for something like psycho-physical parallelism. But you can conceive that the soul organization, which is anchored in the warmth ether, is affected by fear and that such fear comes to expression in a change of your warmth state. In that way the warmth organization is transferred to the respiration, to the fluid and as far down as the solid human being. That is the only possibility of building a bridge between the physical and the soul element.

Without gaining such insight into the human being you will never be able to make the transition from the healthy human being, from an understanding of the healthy human being, to insight into the sick human being. Because, you see, if we take some component of the human organization, say the liver or kidney, which under so-called normal circumstances in some way receives its impulses from the I-organization in that these impulses from the I-organization first act on the warmth organism and then pass down into the sharply contoured liver or kidney and so on—if we look at that, then there is of course a possibility that this intervention by the I-organization through the warmth organization is intensified in the organ compared to the normal behaviour. In other words, the I-organization has too strong an effect on the warmth organization with regard to the liver or the kidney in a way that it should not. And given the configuration of the human organism so that the I-organization can work properly within it, this also provides the possibility for the human organism to fall ill if these structures appear in a wrong or, if you like, dislocated way. Because if you think of the human organism in the way that physiologists and anatomists think of it today it cannot fall ill. Where is the illness supposed to come from? There must be some possibility in the organism for the illness to arise. Now the I-organization has, for example, to act on the heart in a certain powerful way, i.e. it has to act on the heart by way of the warmth organization. If circumstances then cause what is supposed to act on the heart through the warmth organization to act on the kidney or the liver—in the external world, too, you can divert warmth states to another location in a detrimental and disharmonious way—then something happens in the organism which must happen there; the only thing is that it has been dislocated and the possibility of falling ill is given.

Only by taking these things into account can you learn to understand how it is possible for us to fall ill, not by any other means. You have to tell yourself that everything which happens in the human organism is a process of nature. But illness is also a process of nature. Where does the healthy process stop and the disease process start? Where is the transition from one to the other? These questions simply cannot be answered if we stop at what we have in anatomy and physiology. Only once you know that what is disease in the liver is healthy in the heart, and is required there if the human being is to be complete, can you learn to understand the possibility of falling ill. Because if the human organism were not able to generate from the I-organization the warmth organization that is required in the heart region then the human organism would not be able to think or feel anything, for example. But if it acts on the liver or kidney organization then it becomes necessary to drive it out of there again, to confine it to its original limits, we might say.

And you see, there are substances and substantial activities out there in nature which can take on for each organ the activity of the etheric body, the astral body and the I-organization. Say, for example, that the I-organization acts in an incorrect way on the kidney—this is all by way of an introduction today (we will talk about these things in a more technical way in the next few days)—let us say the I-organization in the kidney acts too strongly, the kidney is given the opportunity to do what the I-organization would normally do in this abnormal sick state by administering *Equisetum arvense*. So you have the situation that when the kidney is sick, the I-organization acts on it in such a way as it should act on the heart and not the kidney. There is activity there which should be somewhere else and which exists because the I-organization intervenes too strongly. You can only remove that activity if you artificially introduce another activity that is equivalent to this activity of the I-organization. That is what you can introduce to the kidney if you succeed in administering the function, the activity of *Equisetum arvense* to the kidney in the right way. The kidney has a great affinity with *Equisetum arvense*. In an instant its activity is transferred to the kidney and the I-organization is taken out. And once the sick organ can carry out its diseased activity by different means and something like the I-organization can return to its actual task then the I-organization has a healing effect. You can call on the so-called higher bodies for a healing action if you drive them out of the sick organ and return them to their task. Then the body concerned will indeed have a healing effect on the sick organ. But if you want to penetrate as far as the forces which exist, if you wish to learn to know the human organization in its relationship to the way that the cosmos is configured, to the way that the three realms of nature are configured which surround the human being on earth, then you have to pursue a science that is different from the science often practised today.

Let me give you an example. You all know what an ant heap is like. You know that you get formic acid from ants. Chemists or, indeed, pharmaceutical chemists, talk about formic acid in the way they do but they are not aware of the following. They do not know, for example, that a forest in which ants do not do their work produces terrible harm through what rots away in the roots and so on, produces terrible harm with regard to earth development. We might say that the earth perishes from its rotting organic residues. But imagine wood—and I speak here in broad terms by way of introduction—from which the vegetation has been removed, which has gone over into a kind of mineral state, has become pulverized, rotten. The activity of the ants means that there is always formic acid in an exceptionally high potency in the ground and the air in forests. The formic acid penetrates the rotten wood and as a result future development is safeguarded so that the dust does not dissipate into space but can provide material for the further development of the earth. Thus such substances which appear to be nothing more than excretions of insects or other animals actually safeguard the further development of the earth if their function is properly understood.

You see, examining substances in the way that chemists do today never leads to an understanding of the cosmic tasks of the substances. But without understanding the cosmic tasks of the substances it is impossible to understand the tasks of the substances which are administered internally to human beings. The thing which happens quite unobtrusively with formic acid outside in nature also happens continuously with formic acid within the human organization. As I already emphasized in another lecture,[2] the human organism is dependent on having a certain amount of formic acid within it as the formic acid restores the human substance which otherwise falls prey to the ageing process. We might note in certain circumstances that a person has too little formic acid in his or her organism. But what you have to know is that the various organs have different quantities of formic acid in them. Now it is a matter of discovering that a person has too little formic acid in an organ and then administering formic acid to that organ. You will find cases in which formic acid is administered in which it does not help at all, other cases where it helps a great deal. It can happen that the organism directly resists the administration of formic acid but that it is quite willing to make formic acid from oxalic acid if the oxalic acid content is raised. In cases where the administration of formic acid does not help it is often advisable to give oxalic acid because oxalic acid turns into formic acid in the human organism. That is just an indication of the necessity to be familiar not only with the firmly contoured organs but also in detail with the fluid process—and not just in the human organism but also in the cosmos.

You see with regard to certain processes in nature caused by human beings we can observe them but their full meaning cannot be understood through a natural scientific interpretation.

Let me illustrate a very simple phenomenon. There are fig trees in southern regions. There are fig trees which in the first instance produce wild figs and fig trees which produce particularly cultivated figs which are sweet. The people are very sophisticated in the way they produce the sweet figs. They do the following: they cause a certain type of wasp[3] to lay its eggs in the fig, in a normally grown fig. The egg turns into a grub which pupates. Now this process is interrupted by these people and in a second run the young wasp generation is induced to lay eggs. In this way, by a second lot of eggs being laid by the generation which was produced in the same year, a considerable sweetness is produced in the fig in which the eggs from the second generation were laid. The people in the south do this by taking general figs which are almost ripe and tying two together with raffia so that they hang from the branch. The fig is tapped by the wasps, considerably speeding up the ripening of the fruit because it has already been cut off. As a result the first wasp generation also develops very fast, goes over to the other fig, which has not been picked, and it is made significantly sweeter as a result.

This process is very important, my dear friends, because in nature itself, in the developing substance of the fig, the same thing is happening in a compressed form which happens in an extended form when the wasp or, indeed, a bee takes the nectar from the flower, carries it to the nest or hive and produces honey. The extended process from the flower, whose nectar the bee collects and takes to the hive, to the production of honey in the hive takes place in the fig itself. The people in southern regions trigger the honey producing process in the fig by making the young wasp generation tap the fruit. This fig, which has been injected by the young generation, gets a honey-producing process in it. You have here the metamorphosis of two processes of nature, one of which is extended in that the bee takes nectar from distant flowers and produces honey from it in the hive. The other one takes place on the same tree on which the two figs are suspended which ripen more quickly, where the wasp generation develops more quickly and injects another fig. Because other figs are injected, sweet figs appear everywhere. Such processes should really be studied because those are the processes of nature which are important. Processes take place in human beings of which physiologists and anatomists today simply have no idea because they do not extend their observations to such processes of nature as I have just described. It is important to observe particularly the finer processes in nature because that is the way to achieve a real understanding of the human being.

But all of these things require a real feeling for nature, being able to see the connection between warmth, air currents, air warming up and cooling down, the action of the sun's rays on warming or cooling air, moisture in the atmosphere, the wonderful play of the dew in the morning on flowers and plants, the wonderful processes which take place in an oak apple, let us say, which also arises as the result of a wasp sting and the deposit of an egg. You do have to be able to observe these things with a macroscopic eye. That requires a feeling for nature. And there is most certainly no feeling for nature present if everything is made dependent, as happens in today's observations, on the exclusive focus on the preparation that comes with use of the microscope. You simply remove the whole thing from nature. You see, a terrible illusion exists in this respect. What do we actually want to achieve when we use a microscope? We want to see what we cannot see with the naked eye. By magnifying the object, we think it will have the effect it has when it is tiny. But we are looking at a quite false object, an untrue object. Using a microscope only makes sense if you have enough of a feeling for nature for you to be able to modify the object inwardly to its correct small size after having looked at it in the microscope. Then it is a different matter; you see something quite different. If you see something that has been magnified, you must be able to reduce it in size again within yourself simply through your inwardness. Most people do not do that. People mostly do not have any idea that the magnitudes of natural objects are by no means relative. The theory of relativity[4] is something beautiful and magnificent and beyond dispute for most areas—except the human organism! Three years ago I took part in an academic discussion. Those people did not have the faintest idea when they were told that the human organism cannot, for example, be twice the size it is, it would not be able to exist. The size it has is determined by the cosmos in a way that is not relative for it but absolute. And if it is too large, as in gigantism, or too small, as in dwarfism, we are dealing with medical conditions. And so we have to say that when you see something under the microscope you are in the first instance looking at a lie and you must be able to reduce it to the truth. But you can only reduce it to the truth if you have a feeling for nature, for what is happening in nature.

Under those circumstances it is important to be able to look at a beehive and learn that the individual bee is stupid. It has instincts but it is stupid. But the beehive as a whole is exceptionally wise. We recently had quite an interesting discussion up there with the workers for whom I give a lecture twice a week. We had discussed the realm of the bees[5] and in that connection a question arose which is very interesting. Beekeepers know its importance very well. If a beekeeper who is well liked by his bee colony falls ill or dies the whole of the colony really does descend into disorder. That is so. Well, one person whose thinking was right in line with current views said: 'But bees cannot see that well, they have no idea about the beekeeper. How is some sort of common bond supposed to arise? What's more, let us assume the beekeeper looks after the beehive in one year and the next year there is a completely different bee colony in it, it is completely new apart from the queen, there are lots of young bees. How is the common bond supposed to arise in that situation?' I answered as follows: 'Anyone who knows anything about the human organism knows that it replaces all its substances within a specific period. Let us assume someone gets to know another person who goes to America and comes back ten years later. It will be a completely different person to the one whom he knew ten years ago. All the substances are different, the assembly is completely different. That is no different to what happens in a beehive in which the bees have been replaced but the common bond between the beehive and the beekeeper is maintained. Such a common bond is based on the enormous wisdom which exists in the beehive. It is not just a heap of individual bees but the beehive really does have a concrete soul of its own.'

That is something which in turn has to be included in our feeling for nature, the view that the beehive has a soul. We will then be able to transfer such views, which are supported by a real feeling for nature, to all kinds of other things. And only such knowledge, which is supported by a feeling for nature which not only knows how to use a microscope but also a macroscope, if I may use such a term, will allow us to penetrate as far as the healthy and sick human being. That is what we will do in the next few days, and in doing so we will take account in particular of those things which I refer to as morality in medical studies and medical science. That is what we will do in the next few days.

LECTURE 2

DORNACH, 3 JANUARY 1924

MY dear friends,
As we are now considering using the eight hours after all, I can proceed
a bit more slowly than I could have done if we had been in a hurry. That
is undoubtedly of benefit.

Now today I would like to continue the material from yesterday in
such a form that I tell you about the specific characteristics of the
individual components of the human being. As you know, I drew your
attention yesterday to the fact that we can only look at the whole
human being in such a way that we distinguish the physical body and
connect it with all those things which have fixed contours in the human
being. Then we have what I would like to call the fluid organism. This
fluid organism is permeated by the forces of the etheric body which,
however, connect with the physical body as some kind of original
components. The fluid human being is permeated by the etheric forces.
These are the peripherally acting forces, the forces which are active from
everywhere. Then we have the astral body, which we have to consider in
such a way that a spatial way of looking at it is completely insufficient.
We have to be clear that we have to look at the astral body in purely
qualitative terms; a quantitative view is no use at all. We have to think
of it as residing in a world which is not a spatial world as we know it but
which lies outside this spatial world.

And that applies even more so when we consider the I-organization.
Now the matter will most easily become clear if we start with the I-
organization. What does it represent? The I-organization is perceived in

the physical world in the form of the physical body. It can of course only be perceived in the physical world in the inner and outer form of the physical body. But when we look at the human physical body we must be clear that the way in which it exists in the physical world has nothing whatsoever in common with the forces acting in the physical world. Because at the moment that the human being passes through the portal of death, when the I-organization leaves the physical body, that is the moment when the physical body starts to become subject to the forces of the external world. But that means that it is destroyed, not that it is built up. If you consider that the physical body is destroyed by the forces which are in external nature, you cannot but realize that it cannot be subject to the forces of the physical world in any way in its form. So if the I-organization forms the physical body, that means that it removes it from the forces which are otherwise found in the earthly human environment.

In other words, the I-organization is something quite different to what we find in the physical world. Now it is the case that the I-organization is related, truly related, to death. That means that what happens suddenly with death takes place continuously during earth life through the I-organization. Human beings actually die continuously except that this dying is balanced out. In order to be able to picture the situation, think of yourself faced with the Penelope problem* in reverse. Imagine you are occupied each day with shovelling away a pile of earth near your house and during the night, when you are not present, someone shovels it back again. And for as long as the pile can be shovelled back you have to shovel it away. But once this pile begins to get smaller through the activity of the person who is shovelling it back, there is less and less to do until it has disappeared completely, at which point there is no longer anything there for you to do. That is approximately the relationship of the I-organization to the

---

* In order to stay faithful to her husband Odysseus, and wanting to resist the advances of the many suitors who are seeking to take advantage of Odysseus' long absence in the Trojan War, Penelope tells them that she is weaving a burial shroud for Odysseus' father Laertes and will make her choice once she has finished. Every night for three years she unravels part of the shroud again until her trick is revealed to the suitors by an unfaithful maid.

physical body. When you give food to the physical body you provide it with substances from the earthly environment. These substances which you provide have their inner forces, have a certain configuration of forces. And when you eat table salt, for example, as an additive for food, then this table salt, because it comes in from the outside, has the real inner urge to be active which it has externally as table salt. However, as soon as it gets into your mouth you start to deprive it of these characteristics and then to remove more and more of them so that finally, if the I-organization is sufficiently at work, there is nothing left in you of the table salt as it is on the outside. The table salt has become something completely different. The activity of your I-organization consists precisely in transforming the food you eat. When you no longer have the possibility in the physical body to take in food, then the I no longer has a task just as you no longer have a task if no one shovels a new pile of earth next to your house. The inability to absorb food means that it is impossible for the I to work in the physical body through the warmth conditions. We might say that death is the result when it is no longer possible to transform the outer substances such that they do not retain anything of what external substances have but are wholly in the service of the I-organization.

What does the I-organization actually do in the physical body? It destroys it constantly, it does the same thing that death does, with the exception that this is always balanced by the physical body being able to assimilate external substances as food so that you have the polar opposition between I-organization and food. But for the human being the I-organization means the same thing—only in an ongoing, continuous activity—as death means in a single event, in condensed form. You are constantly dying through your I-organization, i.e. you are destroying your physical body in an inward direction whereas external nature destroys your physical body from the outside when you pass through death. The physical body can be destroyed from two directions and the I-organization is simply the sum total of the destructive forces in an inward direction. We might well say that the I-organization has the task of bringing about death—we will see later why that is so—but in the first instance it does really appear as if the I-organization has no other task than continuously bringing about death in the human being. And this is only ever prevented by new food so that the work of bringing about death is only ever in its beginnings. So we have the situation that the I-organization is actually qualitatively identical with death and the physical organization is actually identical with food. So much just in outline initially, we will discuss it in greater detail later.

> I-organization   = Death
> Physical organism = Nourishment
> [Plate 2]

These two processes, which are at work in the human being as polar processes, have the astral body and the etheric body between them. You see, the astral body only works directly into the aeriform part of the human organism and from there by way of the etheric body on the fluid organism and the nutritional or physical organism. We have the reciprocal connection between the etheric and astral organism in each individual human organ. If we look at the effect of the etheric organism on any organ, the effect can be seen in that the organ obtains burgeoning, budding life. Everything that is vitality in an individual organ or the organism comes from the etheric organism.

If we look at the astral organism, it always has the tendency to paralyse burgeoning, budding life—not to kill it but to paralyse it. The I-organization endeavours continuously to kill the organism and the individual organs, and that must be countered by something that gives vitality to the organs and stimulates them like the nutritional substance ingested from the outside, something that is particularly active in the childhood and youth of human beings.

The etheric impulses are opposed by the activity of the astral body which continuously paralyses etheric activity. Let us assume that there was only etheric activity in your organism, burgeoning, budding life: you would never develop a soul life, never be able to develop consciousness. You would have to vegetate along in a plantlike existence. Everything wants to grow and sprout but no consciousness is developed in growth and sprouting. In order for consciousness to develop there has to be a certain paralysis of the etheric burgeoning and sprouting life. And as a result we have the continuous beginning of illness in any organ that is subject to a certain amount of such paralysis, even in a person's ordinary life. You could not develop consciousness without continuously developing the tendency to fall ill. Because if you wanted to be nothing but healthy you could do that but you would have to vegetate. If you wish to develop a soul life, if you wish to develop consciousness, you have to begin with the vegetating part but then you have to paralyse it to a certain extent. And thus the etheric and astral organisms stand in polar opposition, not as much as the physical organism and I-organization but once again in a weaker sense whereby the astral organism must to a certain extent continuously paralyse what is effected by the etheric organism. Hence what the astral organism does each day in the life of human beings is truly a continuous tendency towards illness. What the etheric organism does is bursting with health. And you can say—just as we can abstractly say that the human being consists of physical body, etheric body, astral body and I-organization—that the human being consists of nutritional processes, of burgeoning and sprouting health-giving processes, as well as of continuous processes of illness and of something which is a process of continuous killing, of arrest, until the killing processes are summed, form an integral, as it were, and death occurs.

Take this astral organism which continuously has the tendency to make an organ or the whole human being ill in some way. Of course you only need to observe yourself in a truly healthy way to see that this is how things are because you could have no feelings if you did not have the astral organism. Just think of it like this: we have the etheric organism through which life develops; we have the astral organism which paralyses. Now when we are awake—I will come to sleep later—there must be a continuous back and forth in a fragile balance between the etheric and the astral. That is what gives human beings feelings. They would not feel anything if this back and forth did not exist. But now imagine that the astral activity is not immediately beaten back by the etheric activity. If it is beaten back, if the astral activity is rejected immediately by the etheric as it arises, normal feelings are produced. We will see on a physical level how this is connected with the activity of the glands. But if the astral organization becomes more powerful so that the organ cannot respond sufficiently in its etheric activity, then the organ is taken hold of too strongly by the astral activity. Instead of there being a back and forth, the organ becomes deformed; the astral body contains the source of illness simply through the fact that it has caused greater paralysis than it should do, i.e. that there has been no rebalancing. And illness is in reality connected in such a way with the feelings that we can say that human feelings are simply a reflection in the soul of illness. When the back and forth takes place, the same process underlies the feelings at the moment when they arise which indicates a disease process if the astral element gains the upper hand. The situation can also arise, however, that the astral is left behind and the etheric gains the upper hand. Then there is excess growth, i.e. illness in the other direction. If we see the dominance of the astral in inflammatory states, we can see the dominance of the etheric in the appearance of excessive growth. And so we must say that in the normal life of feelings there is a constant fragile balance between excessive growth and inflammatory processes. Normal human life needs the possibility of becoming ill. But there has to be a continuous balance. You see, this allows for the possibility of being able to see a lot in the feeling life of the human being which represents pathological processes, provided we have learnt to see it properly. If we are able to observe such things, we can see the approach of an illness a long time before it can be diagnosed physically when the feeling life no longer functions properly. Illness is nothing more than the abnormal feeling life of the human being.

The feeling life remains in the soul element because there is a constant balance in the etheric. As soon as the balance no longer takes place, the feeling life penetrates down into the physical body, combines with the body. As soon as the feeling life infiltrates the organs, illness appears. So if a person can under normal circumstances maintain his or her feelings in the soul, he or she remains healthy; if he or she cannot do that, the feelings infiltrate down into the organs and illness arises.

I say that by way of introduction so that you can see how important it is for a physician to have a sharp eye also for the human soul life. And basically it is not possible to develop a feeling for diagnosis if we do not have a sharp eye with regard to the soul life. We will look at that in detail later and explain it further.

But what is the situation if we include the I-organization and physical organism in our considerations? Let us first look at the nutritional process. This nutritional process constantly destroys the substances of the external world. The astral organism paralyses what the human being is inside through the etheric organism; an inner balance is created between the astral and the etheric organism. A balance is created between the I and the physical organism, between the external and the internal world, so that we can say that salt, as we know it, is external world. If salt is taken hold of by nutrition and the I-organization, the I-organization must be in a position to leave nothing of the salt as it is outside but everything must be transformed. If anything is left over, that represents a foreign body in the human organism. But you must not just see such foreign bodies as something with defined contours— that is least frequently the case. Such a foreign body can also be external warmth. You must not have any warmth in the organism which you have not processed yourself through the I-organization. Imagine a human being, and in this human being you experience that he or she is taken hold of in some way by an external warmth state which he or she has not worked on just like a piece of wood is taken hold of by an external warmth state. This external warmth state is not just a stimulus in order to create its own warmth as a reaction, as an effect, but the external warmth—or coldness—directly affects the human being. Then we can say: the inner balance between illness and health is triggered by the astral and etheric organism, the balance between the human being and the world through the polar opposition between the physical body and I-organization.

It is important to be able to see how these four components of the human organism work. As you can see, it is not possible to recognize an illness from the external physical organism. That which is illness takes place wholly in the supersensory sphere. We have to have an understanding of the astral organism if we want to gain any understanding of illness. And you will understand this from another fact, even if we are still talking in superficial terms today by way of introduction. Pain can occur in an organ. If the astral body becomes too powerful, the organ is deformed and pain occurs. If the organ immediately balances the influence of the astral body as it arises, feelings are produced. But pain is basically feeling, just intensified feeling arising from such deformation so that we can understand why pain always accompanies phenomena of disease. Otherwise we might very well ask why pain occurs at all when we become ill. We can understand very easily why pain occurs if we know that the illness is only present in feelings which become so intense that this feeling life has a deforming effect on the organ. You will see that all phenomena related to feeling can truly be assessed from the intense observation of the human soul life. But we can really only see these things in the right light if we tell ourselves that it makes a difference in human beings, of course, if one or another organ is taken hold of by the excessive activity of the astral body. Let us assume, for example, that the liver is taken hold of by the astral body. The liver behaves differently, quite differently, from other organs. It can be deformed to a high degree by the astral body without pain being caused, without pain arising directly in the liver as an organ. That is why liver disease is so hidden, so sly, because it does not announce its presence by pain. The reason for this is that the liver is the organ which by nature of its whole constitution represents an enclave in the human organism. Processes take place in the liver which of all the processes occurring in the human organism are most similar to those in the external world so that in fact human beings are human to the least extent in the liver. They become external world, have a section of external world inside them. That is very interesting. We have the external world [see drawing], we have the human being and in the human being we have, in turn, a section of external world. It is almost as if a kind of hole had been

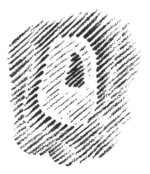

See also Plate 2

punched into the human organization. And just as it would not hurt if the astral body were to imprint itself on this piece of cloth, it would not hurt either if the astral body imprinted itself on the liver. The astral body can destroy but it cannot hurt as far as the liver is concerned because the liver is the organ which is excluded, through which a section of external world appears in the human organism like an enclave.

You will never understand the human organism unless you are prepared to look at these things. You will find a wealth of information about the liver in the physiological and anatomical literature. You will understand it if you know that the liver is the organ inside human beings which is most foreign to them. And why is the liver inside human beings most foreign to them? If you look at the human eye—or any sensory organ—it is like a cavity which goes from the external world into the human being. There are processes in the eye which we can almost understand with physics. With the eye it is actually quite simple to be nothing more than a physicist with regard to the human being. You draw a picture, make a few lines—which are actually terrible nonsense—which illustrate the process of the refraction of light and the way the image is produced in a normal lens. People then use exactly the same drawing for the eye. They draw a ray of light which goes through the lens and is refracted, forms an image at the back of the eye and so on. People have become quite the physicist with regard to the eye; and since the time of Helmholtz the ear has almost become a piano.[6] So the view which applies to external nature has become quite widespread with regard to the sensory organs. Something continues from the outside to the inside. A section of external world continues to the inside. That is indeed justified in terms of developmental history. You can see in certain lower animals how the eye has been formed from the outside through being turned to the inside and being filled from the outside, so that the eye is folded into the organism, we might say, and does not grow out of it. Thus we have a section of external world in the organism in the sense organs. But they are open to the outside; the external world enters the organism through the sense organs like an inlet. Now the liver is enclosed on all sides but it is like a sense organ, a sense organ which, indeed, displays great sensitivity in the unconscious with regard to the nutritional value of the individual substances we take into us.

And we have to say that we will only understand what takes place in the digestion, in nutrition, if we do more than only ascribe to the liver those physical processes which are frequently ascribed to it today. They are only an expression of the soul and spiritual element. We have to see the liver as being an inner sense organ for the nutritional processes. And as a result it is much closer to the earthly substances than our normal sense organs. With the eye we are in the first instance exposed to the effect of the ether, with the ear to the air; the liver is directly exposed to the material qualities of the external world and has to perceive these material qualities.

The heart is another sensory organ. But while the liver is exposed with its perceptive capacity to the external substances entering the human being, the heart is a sense organ for perceiving the whole of the interior of the human being. It is an absurdity—as you might have seen from some of the presentations I have given—that the heart is a kind of pump[7] which drives the blood through the arteries. The movement of the blood is caused by the I and the astral body. And in the heart we merely have a sense organ which perceives the circulation, namely perceives the circulation from the lower to the upper human being. So, you see, the liver must see in the digestive process the value of, say, some carbohydrate in the human being. The heart must see how the astral body and I work in the human being. Thus the heart is a wholly spiritual sense organ, the liver a wholly material sense organ. That is a distinction we have to make. We must come to a qualitative under-standing of the organs. How does the natural science on which medicine is based proceed today? Tissue is casually taken from a part of the organism, let us say the heart or liver. This tissue is examined for its external physical structure and consistency. But that says nothing whatsoever about the organ concerned in the human organism. I have a knife here and a knife here and I examine them. This one and that one. If I investigate them by their form, what the knife looks like, blunt edge at the back, cutting edge at the front, inserted in a handle, I only discover that this is a knife and that is a knife. I have to move on from this kind of examination, I have to relate the object to a whole and then I can find the difference between a steak knife and a kitchen knife. Looked at externally, a kitchen knife could also be used as a steak knife.

I cannot, therefore, recognize just through the outer shape whether I am dealing with a kitchen knife or a steak knife but have to look at each thing in its context. Similarly I cannot learn anything about the importance of an organ if I just look at it in the way that is done today; I always have to look at it in its complete context. Merely investigating the structure and composition of an organ is useless.

People are terribly naive in this respect today. A certain physiological institute conducted experiments on how mice could be fed on milk. They can be nourished very well. They do exceedingly well. They become large and fat. Now to prove that there was something else in the milk in addition to its components, the components were taken separately and fed to the mice. These experiments were carried out. The mice perished in three or four days; they could not be kept alive. What did these people do? They said: so the milk not only has components we know about, it has another substance, the vitamin. They had to assume another very fine substance, the vitamin. They invented such a substance. But that is not the point. The point is that when you have the components of milk it is as if someone said: here we have a watch with a chain, I then learn about the gold, the silver, the other metals in the watch, the glass and so on. Well, the glass, gold, silver, the other metals do not yet make a watch. The watch lies in what the watchmaker's idea makes of them. And in the case of the milk and its components the idea of the watchmaker is that the components contain the earthly qualities, the qualities which the individual components have from the earth. Alongside these components the peripheral forces are also present up to a certain time, which come from the etheric body.

We have to decide finally to accept these things as existing. It really has nothing to do with concealment that things are invented, but stuff like the vitamin is an invention which simply establishes what is there. A quite different way of looking at things must gain ground.

If you eat too many potatoes, you will not manage to establish the effect of the potato on the human organism by determining the quantity of carbohydrates; that will be of no use whatsoever. The other carbohydrates which are present in leaves, for example, and not in the rhizome, or in fruit if you will, they are processed in the digestive tract. The potato is something quite unusual. It enters the human organism with its forces to such an extent that what happens with beans in the digestive tract does not happen with potatoes until the brain. Nutritional processes continuously take place in the brain, too. I just want to indicate these things in order to explain them in greater detail later. So someone who eats too many potatoes may be asking too much of his or her brain. He or she transfers processes into the brain which should take place below the brain. This gives us the possibility to gain something from medicine with regard to our hygiene, with regard to the whole of social life as such, by learning in this way to find out something about the relationship of the human being to the surrounding matter not from its chemical consistency but from the global context.

There is a fundamental difference between a substance occurring in the leaf or the rhizome. It is much more important to know from which part of the plant it comes than whether it contains carbohydrates. The rhizomes are more connected with the head organization of the human being, the flower and leaf organizations more with the lower human being. And a totally unimportant role is played by the chemical consistency. You have to understand the relationship between human beings and their environment on the basis of quite different things if you want to make a proper judgement about what is healthy and what is pathological, i.e. the real substance of the illness and its medicine. Taking account of the indications provided by abstract chemistry is something which has gradually undermined any knowledge of the human being because by knowing the chemical consistency of something you do not know the real relationship between human beings and their environment.

Take another example. The way of looking at things obtained from chemistry alone shows that oxygen is necessary in the air but nitrogen not to the same extent. And we might think, based on the way that people think about oxygen and nitrogen today, that it is not so important with regard to the breathing if some air has too little nitrogen as long as there is enough oxygen. But it turns out that when there is too little nitrogen in the air the human being gives off nitrogen[8] to replace it in the surrounding air.

Human beings are dependent on there being a certain relationship between their own nitrogen content and the nitrogen content in the surrounding air, quite apart from the breathing.

All these things are of great importance for an understanding of the human being. But all these things, although they may be researched or perceived by the occasional person, remain fruitless for today's scientific world if the foundations do not exist for integrating the human being into his or her environment. That is what we intend to do in our considerations in order thereby to throw a light on the healthy as well as the sick human being.

I-organization	=	Death
Astral organization	=	Illness
Etheric organization	=	Health
Physical organization	=	Nutrition

LECTURE 3

DORNACH, 4 JANUARY 1924

M_Y dear friends,
Let me tell you that from tomorrow we will do this in such a way that you consider the questions you would like to ask and then give me those questions or write them down for me, so that in the course of the lectures I can take account of all your wishes so that all the things you want to raise are raised.

Now today I still want to tell you something which is directly related to our reflections yesterday about human beings themselves and their relationship with the world. It is of no use if here, in an anthroposophical reflection on the human being, we are embarrassed, as it were, in front of those who have views about the human being based on present-day science—actually have non-views about the human being—and if we try to diverge as little as possible from the things which are generally accepted. Because it is the case that in major and significant things the truth diverges considerably from what is accepted today. The truth diverges exceptionally strongly from what is generally accepted today. And thus anyone who strives for the truth today will also have to have the courage to understand things which are thought of by current science as exceptionally absurd. Nevertheless, it is necessary—not here, but elsewhere—that you should concern yourselves with this kind of present-day external science if you truly want to make people healthy, if you want to mix, as it were, with those who heal from such a perspective of the external world, that you should concern yourself with such external science in a way which I will go on to explain. Because otherwise you will be forced to stumble about with the truth among the errors of the present day.

The matter at hand is considered today as if we were dealing with 70 or 80 substances on earth[9] with specific forces at work in them, attracting and repelling forces and so on, forces which act through specific equivalent numbers, atomic weights and so on. You then get to certain so-called laws of nature with which the attempt is made to create an overview as to how the substances are formed, how they conform with the laws of nature, and then people build a fantasy construct of what the human being is supposed to be, based on the various forces whose origin is sought in the substances and so on. But it is not like that. Human beings are most certainly not subject only to the influences which come from earthly substances either in their form as a whole or in the forces which sustain their nutrition and growth. We have already seen when we were considering the etheric body that it is most certainly under the influence of forces which stream in from the periphery, from the cosmos. If you now look at these two types of force, the forces which come from the substances of the earth and the forces which come from the periphery, you already have the given situation that each organ requires compensation, a balance, the harmonization of these two types of force. The individual human organ systems vary considerably in the way that such a balance is established.

And let us consider the human head from this perspective. Here we first of all have to note—as I have often done in my lectures where that has been relevant—how the weight which has to be considered in its context in every physical body, how the weight of the brain making up the main weight of the human head is actually largely eliminated because the sharply contoured brain floats in the cerebrospinal fluid. So that we can say that the brain floats in the cerebrospinal fluid which circulates through the spinal canal. If we weigh the brain, it has a weight of 1300 to 1500 grams. But in humans it does not weigh that much, 20 grams at most. Why is this so? Because it floats in the cerebrospinal fluid and according to the Archimedes[10] principle a body loses as much in weight as the weight of the water it displaces. The brain experiences buoyancy in the fluid so that actually only 20 to 25 grams of its weight remains. That is the downward pressure of the brain. If it were to exert a downward pressure of the whole of its weight then there could be no network of blood vessels below the brain because it would be completely squashed; so we can say that it really does apply that the physical characteristic of weight is removed from the brain. Our brain does not live with the physical characteristic of weight but with the characteristic which wants to remove itself from the earth, with buoyancy which opposes physical weight. As regards our head, we are only attracted to the earth with a very small force.

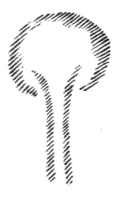

See also Plate 3

That is the one thing. We can see from this that the earthly nature of the brain simply disappears to a large degree through the way that the human being is organized. The human organization is set up in such a way that the earthly forces simply disappear. But that is also the case to a much greater degree. Humanity knows about buoyancy through the Archimedes principle although in a technical respect it is not always taken into account. Otherwise such things as the devastation caused by the reservoir in Italy,[11] where the failure to recognize the Archimedes principle to its full extent was a technical defect, would not have happened. I do not know whether humanity is aware of that, but you could see it in great detail from the descriptions which were made. People consider those laws to be correct which suit them. They ignore those laws which do not suit them.

Now this is not something that only happens in the human head, that weight is lost through the way it is inwardly structured. Something else happens through the special set-up of the human respiratory process, through certain static relationships which occur between inhalation and exhalation. The breath which happens when we breathe in is refracted in a certain way and the opposing breath when we breathe out behaves similarly. Both behave in a similar way to weight and buoyancy, so that the curious thing is that in reality when we walk we leave our head, the brain, at rest with regard to the static relationships. Just as it is not heavy because of the buoyancy of the fluid, a similar thing happens with regard to its inner relationships when we walk. And that applies not just when we walk but in a curious way also with regard to our motion with the earth. We only move with the earth with the rest of our body, not with the brain. For the brain that movement is constantly neutralized so that in a brain weighing 1500 grams only 20 grams remains. Furthermore, it is the case that when we move our head just as fast as the rest of our body it actually remains at rest. It is more difficult to imagine that something which looks to be in motion is in reality at rest than it is to imagine that something which is subject to weight is actually not heavy. But it is nevertheless the case. As far as the inner organization of the human being is concerned, the head is indeed in a position where it is constantly at rest, all the forces are equalized except for a slight downward pressure in a ratio of 20 to 1500, and that there is a very slight forward movement. But essentially the movement is equalized so that we can say that the human head has the same relationship to the rest of the organism—with regard to the inner experience—as a person who sits still in a car and does not move; the car moves and the person makes progress. The human head has the same experience it would have if it were not heavy. It equalizes its motion when a person moves and even the motion of the earth moving with the person.

So there is something very special about the organ of the human head when it excludes, exiles itself from everything that is happening on the earth. The earth is involved only to a small degree in anything that is head activity. On the other hand, the whole of the human head is an image of the cosmos. It is indeed so, that the human head is an image of the cosmos, a real image of the cosmos, and in essence has nothing to do with the forces of the earth. So the way that the brain is inwardly formed is an image of the cosmos and we have an inward shape of the brain whose form we cannot explain with anything earthly but which we have to explain from out of the cosmos. The earth only has an effect by—I say this crudely, but you will understand what I mean—breaching the cosmic formation in a downward direction and inserting into the human being all those things which only have an earthly orientation. You can see that very easily on a skeleton. If you remove the skull you have removed what is an image of the cosmos and you are left with what is half from the cosmos in the structure of the ribs, but they are already under the impression of the earth. Look at the long bones in the legs, the long bones in the arms on a skeleton: these are purely earthly formations. Look at the vertebrae of the backbone on a skeleton, the rough vertebrae of the spine to which the ribs are attached. You have to agree that they have arisen from a state of equilibrium between the cosmic and earthly. And look at the head, there you have a form in the cranial vault in which the cosmos deprives the earth of the possibility of giving shape to itself, a form which is an image of the cosmos. That is how the human forms have to be studied in reality.

But if you study the human forms in this way and also know that the head is at rest with regard to its inner experience, particularly in respect

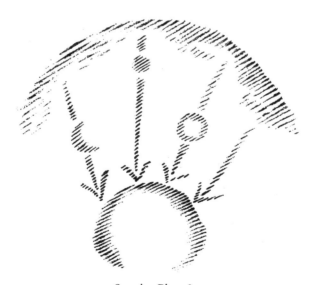

See also Plate 3

of the soft parts, the fluid parts, that it is an image of the cosmos at rest, then you cannot but say that all anatomy and physiology as they are described today are not something you could refer to as the truth because they do not contain the awareness that we are dealing with something which is influenced by the cosmos.

I said there are forces which come in from the periphery as if they were coming in from all sides at the human head. But there is a big difference whether these forces come and are impeded by the moon or impeded by the sun or whether they are impeded by Saturn. The fact that certain stars are present modifies the peripheral forces. The direction from which these forces come is therefore not irrelevant. Their action is significantly modified by the location at which we see a constellation. That is a thought which underlies astronomy in a very amateurish way today, but did so through intuitive wisdom in very early times. No one can have any idea of the way things are in reality from the existing facts today. What I have said is very important for understanding how the human being is formed. Because the fact that human beings are wholly subject to the cosmos in the head, wholly subject to the earth in the long bones of the legs, is also an expression right down into matter of what lies in the formative forces. When you see a human bone structure, you know that it contains calcium carbonate. Then there is calcium phosphate. Both are important for bone structure. Through calcium carbonate the bones acquire their characteristic of being subject to the earth. If the substance of bones was not infused with calcium carbonate the earth could have no effect on bones. Calcium carbonate forms the substantial point of attack for the earth to form the bones in accordance with its formative forces. Calcium phosphate forms the point of attack for the cosmos to form bones. So if you have a long bone such as the human thigh bone, for example, such a thigh bone could not be extended from the top downwards without the action of calcium carbonate. But it would not have the femoral neck without the action of calcium phosphate. That is not altered in any way by the fact quoted by anatomists that the quantity of calcium phosphate and calcium carbonate in the long bone and the femoral neck is not significantly different. Firstly, that is not quite correct if examined in greater detail; they are different. But there is something else to consider in these matters.

The whole of the human organism is designed to have processes which build up and break down. Processes by means of which something is built up and processes by means of which the things that cannot be used for building up are eliminated. A very significant difference between such anabolic and catabolic forces in the substances themselves can be seen in fluorine for example. The ordinary anatomist would say that fluorine plays a role in building up the teeth, it is also found in urine; so we have fluorine here and there. That is beside the point. In building up the teeth, fluorine plays a positive role; the teeth cannot be built up without fluorine. In the urine we find the fluorine which has been removed, which should be broken down. The key thing is to distinguish whether something has been eliminated somewhere and has formed as a result or whether it is absolutely essential for building something up. So that is the situation. If you have a part of a bone which is essentially formed from the cosmos, calcium phosphate works to build it up. In another section of bone calcium phosphate is found as an excretion— and vice versa: in the long bones calcium carbonate builds up the bone but it can be found as an excretion, is eliminated in the direction of the part that has been created out of the cosmos. It has to be said that nowhere is it of relevance whether a substance is present or not; the important thing with regard to its significance in any location in the organism is the direction of its movement.

I once tried to illustrate these things to our friends by saying: let us assume I go for a walk at nine in the morning and see two people sitting peacefully on a bench together; at three in the afternoon I pass by again and the two people are again sitting peacefully together. If I note these two facts I have not done anything because the following situation could be the case. One of the people might have taken a sandwich along and has sat there from nine to three. The other had gone off somewhere and only returned to sit down again shortly before three. The one is rested, the other is tired out. The inner constitution of both is quite different. It cannot therefore be a matter of whether the one or the other person is there, but what did he do, what existential path did he pursue to get there? And thus it is fundamentally irrelevant for an understanding of the human being whether this or that substance is present in an organ. We have to know in what form it is there. Is it there as an anabolic substance or a secretion? Only then can we understand the human being. You will never find the bridge from the quality of a substance that is necessary for the human organism to a medicine if you cannot consider this process properly. Only when you are able to do so will you learn that in fact the distribution of substances in the cosmos is quite different from what people normally think.

It is a striking fact, which people have no longer thought about for as short a period as the last five or six hundred years, that they think certain analytical processes can be used to show that there is iron in the human organism. These processes allow us to say that there is iron in the human organism, in the blood. But you will try in vain to show that there is lead in the human being if the organism is normal. Now we really only know lead in lead ores if present in material quantities. But all the metals which we find in material quantities in the substance of our earth once existed in dissolved, very volatile, even warmth etheric states in their original forms on Saturn, Sun and so on. Now human beings were already present on old Saturn, in a different form of course. They went through all these processes in which iron, for example, has become what it is today from a very volatile, finely distributed, warmth etheric state. They participated in what the world has become and so on. The peculiar thing is that human beings behaved in respect of iron and magnesium in such a way that they integrated them into their own structure. Lead they overcame. They behaved towards magnesium such that they combined the magnesium process with their own process. They behaved towards lead in such a way that they fled from the lead process, they expelled it. So we can see with regard to magnesium that the same forces are at work in the human being as in magnesium externally. Human beings have to overcome them inwardly. But before human beings were enclosed in their skin, when they were still metamorphosing forms which were united with the cosmos, they overcame the lead process so that they still have within them today the surmounting, the expulsion of the lead process. They have within them the anabolic forces of magnesium and the powers to eliminate the lead process.

What does that actually mean? You only need to study what happens to the human organism when it is subject to lead poisoning. It becomes brittle, sclerotic. Hence we could say that the human organism cannot tolerate lead within it. When lead poisoning occurs there is lead in the human organism. However, the organism begins to fight the process which lies in the lead substance—substances are always processes. Lead spreads in the organic process; the organism rises against it and tries to expel the lead. If it manages to do so, it regains its health. If the lead is stronger the organism does not regain its health. The familiar disintegration process associated with lead poisoning occurs in the human organism because the latter can only cope with the processes which overcome the lead process. It cannot have the forces which form the lead substance within it.

If we now investigate what the benefits are to human beings that they have no lead within them, we find the following. You see, human beings are sensory beings in the first instance. They perceive the things around them and then they think about them. They require both things. They must perceive things so that they can establish a connection with the world. They must also reflect, must force back their perceptions and then develop their independence by forcing back their perceptions. If we only perceived, we would always be taken up with external perception. But only by stepping back from things, by reflecting on them, do we become a personality, an individuality. In that way we are not always taken up by things. And if we study the human etheric body it has within it a centre for the forces which reject lead. This centre is roughly where the hair forms its crown. [See Plate 4] That is where the forces which overcome lead radiate out. They radiate into the whole of the organism so that the lead-forming forces can on no account enter the organism. The forces formed by the body which overcome lead are very important because as a result of these same forces I do not remain caught up in the simple observation of this chalk. Otherwise I would indentify myself with what I am looking at. I make myself independent, I paralyse my perception to some extent, but I do so with the same forces which are the forces used to overcome lead so that human beings owe it to the lead-overcoming forces that they can be inwardly unified personalities. The fact that human beings can separate themselves from the world is due to the forces which overcome lead.

It is indeed the case that these forces located in human beings—the existence of which can become quite conspicuous if a certain context, which I will mention shortly, is taken into account—are not just of physical and etheric but also psychological and moral importance. What I mean to say is that human beings take certain metal solids into their body which they combine with their own physical organism, other metal solids they reject. These are only in human beings as processes for repelling, for overcoming. So why does it happen that human beings in the course of their long development from the Saturn period, the Sun period and so on have rejected certain substances which have arisen on the outside and assimilated others? Such rejection at the same time includes the ability of human beings to assimilate independent moral forces within themselves. It is indeed the case that if human beings were inclined to have lead-forming forces within themselves—one could imagine that our present organism does not necessarily need lead but that somewhere it had lead-forming forces, that it contained lead in the same sense that it now has iron—then they would have, as is the case with lead, semi-moral characteristics within themselves in relation to lead. Human beings would have a pathological—today we would call it pathological—affinity to external dirt in the world. Human beings would seek out smelling, stinking substances and smell them to immerse themselves in them. And if we have children and observe how it can happen with children that they have such perverse character-istics—there are children who love to seek out stinking matter, who nibble with their nose on petroleum, for example—then there is always an absence of such lead-repellent characteristics in the blood. Then we have to try and summon this lead-repellent force by clinical or even medicinal means. It is possible to call up this lead-repellent force through forms of treatment which we will discuss later on.

Let us remain with a substance which plays a certain role in the human organism, magnesium. Here we can study a particularly inter-esting thing. I have repeatedly drawn attention to the fact, particularly in the educational field, that the first period of life, which we have to separate clearly from all the following ones, extends as far as the change of teeth. The next period goes to puberty. Now the thing is that just as fluorine is necessary for the development of the teeth, so is magnesium. But the development of the teeth takes place not just in the mouth, the upper and lower jaw, but the whole organism is involved; the magnesium process takes place in the whole organism. And that is of key significance for the human being until the change of teeth. After the change of teeth the magnesium process is no longer of such importance as it was previously because the magnesium forces harden the organism. They coalesce the organism within itself and the concluding point of this consolidation of the human organism, this internal structuring of the forces and substances is concluded with the change of teeth, with the arrival of the permanent teeth. Until that point the use of magnesium is of the very greatest importance for the human organism.

Now the human organism is a whole with regard to its temporal development. It must develop, have magnesium within it. It would not have the proper consolidating forces if it did not have these magnesium processes within it. But it cannot stop producing the magnesium forces. This continues to happen after the change of teeth just as much as it did before. They must be processed in the organism and the key thing after the change of teeth is that the magnesium is overcome, that it is expelled. It moves particularly to the human secretion of milk, it is secreted particularly with milk. Because the secretion of milk is connected with sexual maturity, you can see a peculiar connected process, a periodic process. Take magnesium: until the change of teeth it is consumed, as it were, by the human organism; from the change of teeth to puberty it is expelled and in the forces which form the milk forces magnesium is present as a secretion. Then there is a reversal to the age of 20. Thereafter the magnesium force is used for the finer consolidation of the muscles. Substances are really only compounded processes; lead only appears to be this rough, grey-looking substance. It is nonsense to say that it is a piece of rough substance; lead is a process which takes place within the limits set for the spread of lead—everything is process. We can say that the substantial processes in the human being are not only such that certain substantial processes can be processed in the human being and others are rejected, like the lead process which we will never use and for which we will always need the excretory force. For there are also others, like the magnesium process, which is such that it changes rhythmically so that in rhythmical periods of our life we develop the consuming processes for the magnesium forces and then the excretory processes.

We can see from this that we do not really get anywhere if we only do an analysis and say that the human organism contains magnesium. That tells us nothing at all because at the age of 12 these substances have quite a different meaning than at the age of five or four. And we only get to know the human being when we know that certain substantial processes have a specific relevance in the human organism. If we want to know how the substances that are out in nature continue working in the human organism, then the least important thing is to study the chemical composition of the substances. We have to study something that is hardly studied today at all. If we look at the way substances were studied into the thirteenth and fourteenth centuries, we find the first beginnings of modern chemistry. These beginnings lie in the alchemical processes of the time which often appear silly to us. But there is something else. There was something present at the time which was not developed at all, what today we might call the doctrine of signatures. The doctrine of signatures was particularly used with regard to plants, but also minerals, and it did not see any development.

Take a substance like antimony, stibnite: the particular thing about this antimony is that it has the well-known spiky form, this hairlike form.

If you treat it in a particular metallurgical way you get the antimony mirror when the volatile antimony condenses on a cold surface. In stibnite you have the tendency to make forms which are actually quite clearly forms of the etheric body. What develops there looks very similar to the forms of certain simple plants which nestle up to the etheric body. If we look at the substance of antimony, we have the direct feeling that antimony is very receptive to etheric forces. It nestles in the etheric forces. Everyone can see that by treating antimony electrolytically and connecting it to a cathode under certain conditions. A series of explosions occur which create the transition into the relationships between antimony and the etheric forces. That is a conspicuous case but there was a strong understanding of these things in the past which no longer exists today. We no longer respect such observations as I have indicated. That is why we are in a situation in which we are at a loss with regard to important observations. You see, we have diamonds, graphite, anthracite or mineral coal. All of them are coal, but quite different. Why is that so? If people were really willing to try to understand not just the chemical composition but what in the past was described as the signature, they would begin to understand what a difference there is between mineral coal and graphite. Mineral coal has been created during the Earth process, graphite during the Moon process, the planetary process preceding the Earth, and diamond during the Sun process. And if you look at these things from a cosmic perspective, you will also gain the insight that once again it is not a matter of the substances but of the conditions and periods under which a substance took on a specific, that is a fixed form. After all, if physically real substances are subject to time, time has a specific importance. Because just think, if you take what I have said, you can say that mineral coal is a child, is not yet very old; graphite is a youth, a bit older; diamond is, if not an old man, at least fully adult. If you want to set any task which requires, let us say, mature adulthood, you will not use a child. It depends on the age. So you can see that simply by nature of its cosmic age, coal has a different task wherever it occurs from graphite which is of a more mature age. So it is necessary to look into cosmic processes if we want to learn to understand the relationship between human beings and what is out there in the cosmos. If antimony has a particular affinity with the human etheric body and you introduce antimony into the human organism as a medicine, you have to understand its relationship outside the human being if you want to know what is stimulated in the human etheric body through antimony. You simply have to be willing to go into the finer processes of nature if you wish to understand what any medicine should do in the human being.

LECTURE 4

DORNACH, 5 JANUARY 1924

Now, my dear friends, we have tried to sketch out in the last three sessions the kind of basic knowledge which a physician should try to obtain, knowledge which we could only sketch out briefly as permitted by the short time. But you will have realized that if we wanted to go into detail it would take a long time. This time would, of course, be available on a medical course.

A proper medical course would have to be organized in such a way that an initial part of the course, which would have to comprise at least a year if not longer, would have to be provided for students in which such knowledge is then acquired as the basis of what medicine is all about. I cannot give you more than a kind of outline of what that should be like. And that is why I want you to consider what I have presented in three hours so far as a kind of charcoal drawing of what a physician has to learn. I would like to describe that as the exoteric part of what a physician must know. The next step in the medical course would then have to be the esoteric part of what a physician must know, something which we will speak about now. This esoteric part must build on the basis of the exoteric part. But when you are studying medicine you should on no account disdain to acquire with all seriousness a thorough command of the exoteric part in so far as we can know anything about it. That is difficult in the present time. But as we will see in the sessions to come, a lot can be done in this direction, particularly through the Medical Section in our Dornach School. And it is already possible today to expand what I have indicated in my brief sketch by means of the many details which are available in my cycles and writings. That has only happened to the smallest extent so far and the extension offered by anthroposophical medicine will not come about until the work which I am preparing with the help of Dr Wegman[12] is published in the near future. Then it will be possible to see how anthroposophy can provide a stimulus for medicine and medical studies.

But you must be clear that the study of medicine is a very special course of study which has its own special prerequisites, a course of study in which the findings of spiritual science cannot be ignored. We cannot have a system of medicine in which the findings of spiritual science are not present. The chaotic conditions which we continue to encounter in this field simply exist because a school of thought is setting the tone in medical studies and knowledge which is totally unsuitable for an understanding of medicine. Things are such today that we have a science—including in theology—which is only suitable for technical purposes and not in any way for gaining an understanding of the human being. For you see, real medical knowledge requires something special, which will become clear to you when I speak about how the human being is created.

I already drew attention to it exoterically yesterday, so today and in the following lessons I will make the transition to the esoteric aspect: the external substances are in reality processes. Salt is only the expression of processes; the magnesium processes, iron processes are processes which take place outside in nature. Lead processes, mercury processes are processes which human beings must not have within them, which are outside in nature. But it is only apparently so that human beings do not have these processes within them. How is the human being created? To begin with, the physical base is created through fertilization and this physical base must combine with the etheric body of the human being. But the etheric body is not created through fertilization but is formed around what later becomes the I-organization and astral organization, around the spiritual and soul entity which comes down from the spiritual world and which was present from pre-earthly life. So we are dealing with the actual core of the human being as the spiritual and soul entity which exists, firstly, from earlier incarnations and, secondly, from the time between death and a new birth long before fertilization has taken place. This spiritual and soul core of the human being attaches the etheric body to itself before it establishes a connection with what is created through the fertilization of the physical egg. And the thing which unites with the potential contained in the physical embryo, the I, the astral organization and the etheric organization, this threefold organization unites with what has been created through physical fertilization. You must look at the etheric body as something which is formed from out of the cosmos. Now this etheric body, which is formed out of the cosmos, at the moment when it first unites with the physical organization contains the forces which then do not apply to the physical organization—the lead and zinc forces. It is only apparently the case that human beings are not a microcosm in that they do not contain certain substances. The substances which the human being does not have in the physical body are the most important substances for the constitution of the etheric body so that lead processes, zinc processes, mercury processes and so on indeed take place in the etheric body before it is united with the physical body.

Then the etheric body combines with the physical body—the other parts as well, of course. And the following occurs to a small extent during the embryonic period, but to the greatest extent when respiration starts, that is at birth, when real external respiration starts: then all the forces which the etheric body possesses from the substances which are not based in the physical body are transferred to the astral body and the etheric body takes on those forces which the physical body processes within itself. So the etheric body undergoes a very important metamorphosis, the metamorphosis that it takes on the content, the constitution of the physical body and passes on its own constitution, its affinity with the human environment, to the astral body. The astral body is now intimately connected with what human beings can know. And at the moment, my dear friends, when you start to assimilate not just theoretical knowledge but true, internally digested medical knowledge, at that moment you bring the content to life within you which the astral body already possesses but which has remained unconscious and represents the relationship with the environment.

Let me take a specific case. Take a region, for example, which is melancholy. It is melancholy because the ground in the present constitution of the earth contains gneiss. And the gneiss contains mica which is familiar to you as a mineral. Mica exercises a very strong influence on the local constitution which a human being has in a specific region. Your physical body is different if you are born in a region where there is a lot of mica. It acts on the physical body from the ground, from out of the earth. Now you will find that a lot of rhododendrons grow in regions where there is a lot of mica. The plant can frequently be found in the Alps, in Siberia and so on. Rhododendron substance is intimately connected with the etheric body before it enters the physical body in such regions. This affinity with rhododendrons is passed on by the etheric body to the astral body. So when illnesses occur in such regions which are caused by a preponderance of the action of mica on the inhabitants by way of the groundwater, the etheric body has passed on what it obtained from the rhododendrons to the astral body. That is present externally in the rhododendron plant. From that we can know that there is a sap in the rhododendron which has a healing effect on this illness. That is why in many things, but not in everything, the specific medicine for an illness can be found in the regions in which the parti-cular illness occurs.

Now you have to consider that when you are asleep each night as a physician you immerse yourself in your astral body in the environment that was connected with the etheric body and is now connected with your astral body. When you then acquire medical knowledge, if you know what healing forces exist in the human environment, you experience these healing forces constantly in sleep. In sleep you con-stantly experience confirmation of what you can learn externally through dialectics. And that must be taken into account in any medical course because all external dialectical learning of medical subjects is of no use, is never of use. It becomes dissociated, disordered if the necessary confirmation within the astral body and the environment fails to occur during sleep. Because if the study of medicine is not obtained in such a way that the astral body can say yes to what the physician has learnt in his or her dialogue with the environment, it is as if he or she listened to something which he or she cannot understand, which only confuses him or her. In this way medical knowledge is intimately connected with those things in the life of the human being which lead into sleep. You see, it really is the case that precisely such things must lead to the conviction that medical studies must be acquired by the whole human being, the living, feeling human being. Because something else arises from this nightly intercourse with the healing ingredients which can really never be obtained through dialectical learning: the urge to give real assistance. Without this urge, this feeling of the physician, without the concern for the person who is to be healed, without this urge personally to give assistance there is basically no healing.

You see, here I have to say something that you might find quite strange and paradoxical. But since you do want to learn about what is missing today and what has to come, I have to say this as well because in Dornach we work on the basis of esoteric impulses. You see, I have often been told that it might happen that the medicines we produce—this will appear paradoxical to you but you will have to accept some things as paradoxical—that the medicines we produce in the pharmaceutical laboratory should be carefully protected so that they cannot be copied. I once responded to that by saying that I was not really too concerned about copies being made if we succeeded in introducing true esoteric impulses into our stream. Then people would understand that the medicines are made with an esoteric background, that it is not the same thing if the medicines are made with everything which lives in the esoteric aspect, which is introduced thereby, or if any old factory copies them. That may appear paradoxical to you, but that is how it is. It simply is necessary—much more so than something being done by external means, by commercial tricks—that a certain atmosphere is created which says: there is something behind that which gives these things a healing power based on the spirit. That is not superstition, that is something which, as you will still see, can be thoroughly substantiated through spiritual science. Thus reasonable people will realize that if the medicines that are produced here are taken, it means that a start is being made with what actually needs to be done.

Such objections which have been voiced to me might be the result of people today having no idea that particularly in the medical sphere esoteric, spiritual life has to be taken much more seriously. As soon as you understand this, above all, you will see the real sense—not just formally as happens elsewhere—in which a School, a place to foster medical studies, was to be set up here. You will also understand that the first exoteric medical course should be followed by a second course which approaches the human being in a pre-eminently esoteric way, which immerses medical knowledge in what is an attitude in the human being, a medical attitude.

Certain personalities have always instinctively sought such a medical attitude. And in the last third of the nineteenth century, when actually there was very little of what might be called a medical attitude, one could only see such a medical attitude sporadically produced in individual personalities who were then seen as strange characters. After all, the reputation of the Vienna medical school,[13] with which I really grew up, became so great because essentially this Vienna school took as its basis that part of healing in which therapy is least important, namely pneumonia where one can do least with regard to the central disease, with regard to treatment. That is how therapeutic nihilism, of which you will have heard, arose. Specifically the most important of the Viennese physicians very deliberately defended therapeutic nihilism, i.e. they took the view: medicine does not heal! In a certain sense Virchow[14] also adopted this view. He took the view that of a hundred so-called healed patients one can assume with 50 per cent of them that they would have got better anyway, whether they were given the medicine or not. And with 30 per cent one can say that the medicine was directly harmful. With the remainder, the chosen medicine might have worked by chance. That is not me speaking, that is Virchow speaking, one of the medical giants of the last century. I know illustrious personalities even today who strictly hold this point of view although they might defend therapy. There is no medical attitude in that. But then, the latter cannot be something to which one refers as a mere formality. It must be produced in reality and for that we require the human element in the second course which must build on the exoteric aspect. A human element is required which acts as it did, albeit in a degenerated way, but nevertheless sometimes with what I might call delightful magnificence, in such a personality as Paracelsus.[15] Of course there is a lot one could object to in Paracelsus regarding one or the other point. But he had this medical attitude in a magnificent way. He always knew when he arrived in an area where Rotliegendes[16] was near the surface, came up as earth, that a number of diseases—namely diseases arising from disorders of the blood—were simply due to the fact that the ground contained Rotliegendes. There is a very characteristic development of the pathological process. If you are in an area with much Rotliegendes you will find that the people who have lived there for a long time have become used to the Rotliegendes and display particular characteristics with regard to their temperament. We find that these people have a very active spleen. And if you arrive in that area as a stranger you will find little liking for you; the people are terribly obstinate, self-righteous, naive. They think you are stupid if you question anything they do. That is how it is, the people become used to it in the Rotliegendes. But if a stranger comes who wants to set up a business, he will not tolerate the Rotliegendes, namely the water. He will suffer certain pathological symptoms. Paracelsus says that such diseases which arise there are also passed on to the long-established people there. Paracelsus said: something is surely going on in the sphere of the etheric body; archaeus he called it. Something must surely have happened to the archaeus before it entered the embryo. Now you always find that laburnum grows wonderfully in these regions. You will easily find a sap in laburnum, in the flowers, the leaves, also sometimes in the roots, which can produce a very good medicine, depending on how the human being is constituted.

The point is to obtain a different way of looking at nature as a result of a medical attitude. And so I became acquainted with a physician[17]—I was still a boy at the time—whom you often encountered in the fields and meadows where he communed with the plants, flowers, insects and so on. Three or four luminaries lived in the area where this person worked as a modest physician. We can say that the work of this modest physician, who so loved the flowers of the field, was incomparably more productive for his patients than the work of the state physicians and the other luminaries. Because they obtained their wisdom from school and the things associated with school. But he truly took his wisdom about medicines from his direct contact with nature. But even this only leads to medical knowledge if you can love nature in every detail. You no longer love it when you study it under the microscope. You have to love it, you have to be able to macroscope it. You see, that is where you learn how necessary it is to make this subconscious life of the astral body available for medical knowledge, to make it properly available. Now it is by no means my intention to bring up a whole lot of ancient things but merely to speak about what can be observed in the present. But we simply have to use terminology that has been handed down because language today, including medical terminology, does not have the right terms. Otherwise we would have to invent a terminology. Perhaps it would benefit the spread of our views if we did that. But we would probably have to work on such a terminology for years. And since you would like to hear about it right now, I will use the old terminology with some variations.

It is a good thing if we first look at the plant world—not so much because I want to universally recommend herbal medicines but because we can learn a lot from it and can gain a an immense amount above all with regard to a deeper esoteric view. Now it is of fundamental importance for learning about medicine that we consider three things, but not consider them in the way that our common knowledge and skills are considered today, but really in a different way.

If a student has learnt something today he knows it and thinks: that is good, I know that and can apply it. But the person who is a religiously devout person learns the Lord's Prayer and also gets to know it. But he does not think that it is enough for him to know it and he prays it daily; he prays what he knows. He allows what he knows to pass before his soul each day. That is a completely different view of the matter, something completely different. Or take an initiate. You can assume with some certainty that he is familiar with the elements of esoteric knowledge. He does not care a fig that he is familiar with them, that he has at some point learnt them. It is much more important to him to let the very first elements and the subsequent ones pass through his soul with devotion so that he always gets new momentum in his soul. The religiously inclined person has quite different experiences from the person who only sees something in nature that belongs to the physical world. We always have to find ourselves again in the rhythm of nature if we want to acquire living and not dead knowledge. Knowledge, the activity of knowing, must be rhythmically repeated. That is what I mean when I say that there has to be a medical attitude as the basis for medical knowledge. Obtaining medical knowledge from the nature of the human being and his or her environment is particularly important in a therapeutic respect. It is of particular importance that you note how you let the plants repeatedly pass before your soul.

There are three things in the plant which are of particular importance. The one thing is—and this appears in the plant in a quite wonderful way—the scent of the plant, which is connected with the oils active in the plant. The scent of the plant is the thing that exercises the attraction for certain elemental spirits who want to descend into the plants. And we can, using the terms of the old medicine, truly call this spiritual extract of the plant at work in the scent—which calls forth a kind of longing in the elemental spirits which descend as a result of the scent—the sulphur element of the plant because what underlies the scent in its activity, not in its substance, exists in the mineral sphere in its most concentrated form in sulphur. We can say that even in just observing the sulphur element of the plant we obtain a real understanding of the scent of the plant if we recognize that something spiritual takes place above and below when the plant emits a scent. That is the first thing.

The second thing we obtain is an inner feeling for what grows in the leaf. There are so many opportunities to connect the flowers with the scent of the plant, the leaves with the formal element of the plant. The leaves have such diverse forms: serrated, soft, pointed, blunt, segmented and so on. We should develop a sensitive feeling for this leaflike aspect in the plant because that is how these spiritual beings, who descend through the scent, obtain their vitality. And in that way the endeavour to take on a droplike form radiates in from the periphery of the cosmos. You see, there is something which can give you a wonderful feeling for what is actually contained in the leaf as the form-giving element from the cosmos: namely if you simply develop a love of looking at leaves when in the morning the plants are covered in glistening dewdrops. Because these drops by their nature simply reflect the endeavour of the periphery, the cosmos, to produce the spherical form, the droplike form in plants. It is drops which wholly underlie everything that is leaf in the plant. And if nothing but the peripheral, the cosmic were spiritually active in the plant it would always take on a spherical form. You can see that plants become particularly spherical when the cosmic gains the upper hand, as happens in the way some berries are formed and so on, but also in the way some leaves are formed. But such drop formation is immediately taken over by the earthly forces. The drop is stretched in various directions and a great variety of forms are created. Such striving for a droplike form can be found in mineral concentration in mercury. That is why in ancient medicine such striving to become like a drop was called mercurial. In ancient medicine mercury was not quicksilver but the striving to become like a drop, the dynamic striving to become like a drop. The mercurial is present everywhere where there is this striving to become like a drop. Quicksilver is the metal which takes on a droplike form on earth because the conditions exist for it to do so. Quicksilver has the form on earth which silver has on the moon, where it would also have to be in droplike form. The point is that ancient medicine called everything with a droplike form mercury. All metals were also mercury for the ancient medic. That is something which simply has to be taken into account, that ancient medicine lived in what was flexible, vital. We will have to find our way back to such flexibility, vitality. Then you will have to develop a sense which will make you inclined towards this flexible, vital element to such an extent that you tell yourself: when I walk across the meadows in the morning and see the silvery pearls of dew on the leaves, these silvery pearls of dew will reveal to me what lives in the spirit in the leaves themselves—the striving for the cosmic spherical form. But you have to feel that in order to understand plants. You have to learn to understand them in their spherical form. If you learn to understand plants in such a way that you establish a relationship with their striving for the droplike form and then upwards through the scent, you will gradually acquire a sensitive understanding for everything that acts centrifugally in human beings. Centrifugal forces are at work when human beings cut their nails. They grow again: those are centrifugal forces which pass through the human being. During the first seven years the forces which then reach their conclusion in the permanent teeth are constantly passing centrifugally through the human being. They are expressed to the greatest extent through the formation of sweat. Those things which strive upwards in the scent of the plant and attract the nature spirits also live in the scent of sweat which has a centrifugal direction. So that if you wish to seek what is plantlike in human beings you do indeed have to look in that direction and assume it to be there in its deep striving outwards. In this way you will obtain a deep and intimate understanding of the connection between what is outside and what is inside the human being. For you see, when the etheric body transfers its particular characteristics to the astral body, the whole thing is reversed. The etheric body wants to develop what it takes from the environment upwards. By transferring it to the astral body it develops centrifugally towards the outside [downwards?] so that human beings do indeed carry plantlike development within themselves in this respect.

Look at the plant, how it sinks its roots into the soil, how through the roots it enters into an intimate relationship with the salts in the soil in the widest sense. Here a process takes place which is diametrically opposite to the phenomena accompanying the sensory processes, which are salt processes. Take table salt, which tastes salty in solution, and imagine this process turned into its polar opposite so that the solution is reversed, solidification takes place and the smell and taste become latent. Then you have the process that takes place between the soil and the plant root. That is what is called the salt process in ancient medicine. Ancient medicine did not call the things salt which we do today, i.e. carbonate salts and so on; it called salt what in the plant and the downward pointing root enters into a connection with the substances of the soil. That is the salty element. In constantly directing your attention rhythmically towards these wonderful secrets of nature you are taking practical steps to fill you medical knowledge with life. In other words, you will start, if you try in this way to fill your medical knowledge with life, to look at nature and human beings in such a way that healing comes to you from out of the strong impulse to give assistance of which I spoke to you earlier. It can truly only develop on such a basis—quite specifically. These things must be triggered specifically through assiduous, determined, active exoteric learning, otherwise you will only do muddleheaded things. But it is also necessary to know that the real basis of medical knowledge lies in fact in this rhythmical absorption in the human natural environment, not in theoretical medical learning but in what I have just tried to characterize and what you can live rhythmically.

What I am about to write on the blackboard* is not there for you to know but to keep stimulating in you such vitalization of your medical sense. It goes something like this:

> Healing spirits
> You unite
> With sulphur's blessing
> In the etheric scent;

> You are enlivened
> Through Mercury's striving upwards
> In dewdrops
> In what grows
> In what becomes.

> You stop
> In earth's salt
> Which nourishes the root
> In the soil.

That is what the soul acquires in looking at the environment, awakening the inner sense for what surrounds it. Human beings can then respond:

> I want to unite the knowledge of my soul
> With the fire of
> The flower's scent;

> I want to bestir the life of my soul
> Through the glistening drop
> Of the leafy morning

> I want to strengthen my soul existence
> Through the hardening salt
> With which the earth
> Carefully maintains the root.

Now, my dear friends, what you can acquire through repeatedly

---

* This blackboard has not been preserved.

bringing these things to life in you, like the pious do in prayer, stimulates those forces in the soul which can work medically. Because the normal forces which are used in school today cannot awaken medical knowledge. The latter must be retrieved out of the soul. That is why I always preface the esoteric observations we wish to foster with this: we have to consider how the soul forces first have to be brought to life in order to awaken in the soul those things that lead to medical knowledge.

Lecture 5

Dornach, 6 January 1924

My dear friends,

Following on from yesterday, I have now had a look at your questions. They are all of course connected with the things we discussed yesterday. Now the questions that have been asked, and which comprise what I would like to describe as the first category, have all been raised out of a kind of heartfelt apprehension. Individual questions will find an answer in the course of the lectures. It will not be possible to answer other questions—which are all basically more or less the same—theoretically, except as a result of the things that can arise from this course. Because basically all these questions amount to one thing, namely how the participants in this course can find their medical way after Dornach. These questions will be discussed today, placing them between what I spoke about esoterically yesterday and what I will speak about esoterically again tomorrow with regard to the real continued effect of the impulse which I can only deal with in such a brief way in so few lectures. This real continued effect will in the first instance have to form the basis for what we will continue to discuss esoterically tomorrow.

I want to begin by adding a few things in general which follow on from what was said yesterday. Little is achieved, my dear friends, by generally directing people or by people directing themselves from the sensory and physical world to the spiritual. Such a general reference to the spiritual accords of course in every area of life—and, we have to say, most intensely in the medical field and for physicians searching for their path—with an innermost need which also lives in the soul. But this need is one, in many respects, which must find a greater focus within itself, greater inner clarity, and also (and this is maybe the main thing) greater inner strength than is normally the case. You possess all these things as an inner striving, my dear friends. But a path has to be determined. I can begin by giving the impulse for such a path but you then have to introduce real striving forward in connection with Dornach with this impulse.

Everyone who sets themselves this task—and the questions indicate that this is being done with all intensity—should know that a general striving for the spiritual is not enough. The point is that such striving for the spiritual should take a very concrete form in the various areas of life. And so it is absolutely necessary that we once again immerse ourselves in co-existing with the whole essence of the cosmos, with the reality of the cosmos to a greater or lesser extent. People do not experience the cosmos today and because they do not experience the cosmos they do not experience the spiritual. Because spirituality can only be achieved by way of the cosmos.

The way medical knowledge presents itself through its outer form, its development, its external appearance does not provide any spiritual knowledge about existence. Not until we are able to place things and beings into their complete cosmic context will we be able to look through the veil of nature and see the spiritual forces behind it.

Now it is indeed the case that it was possible in the anthroposophical movement to study, to experience in great detail over the last 20 years the difficulties that can arise when we pursue a spiritual life. And it might at first even look a bit superficial if we outline briefly what those difficulties were. They were simply this, that those who were striving for esoteric things in some area or other simply made it too easy for themselves, refused to make an effort. Quite simply, the esoteric path is a difficult one or it is none at all. And you cannot achieve esoteric development by taking it easy. We have to take the general comment which is made so often, that difficulties have to be overcome, that human beings have first to get beyond themselves, in all seriousness. And from this point onwards, from the time onwards that was initiated by the Christmas Conference in Dornach, a kind of transformation should occur in the whole way that the anthroposophical movement thinks, including in the individual fields. And in seeking your medical path you also have to participate, right from the beginning, in such a real transformation so that the esoteric path is not just some kind of addition but represents nothing less than your life's path being completely filled with esoteric impulses. Everything that can be done in this respect will be done in these lectures. But something has to follow on from that, as I will go on to say at the end of today's discussion.

Let us take another look at something in detail, because if you are not willing, my dear friends, to look at details in spiritual observation, you will not be able to find the path into the spiritual sphere. You should not think that you can truly find the spirit as a dreamer or as someone who indulges in all kinds of vague inspirations and the like. The spiritual must be obtained through real work, with the most serious inner endeavour. And it can only be obtained on the basis of what exists in the spiritual world.

And so, to begin with, let us look at a detail. I have already said that we can learn a great deal from the plant world. But let us now look at such a plant. People today simply see them as the root, the stem, then the flower, the leaves, the pistil in the middle, the stamen and the seeds. The seed develops in the ovaries and people describe what we see in the plant in this way rather like we describe an armchair, with the additional information that sometimes we might also sit in it. That is roughly how people describe plants. They describe how the root is located in the ground, how it absorbs physical forces, chemical forces and substances, how the sap rises through capillaries or similar things. It is considered an error, as false, if we refer to a spiral arrangement of the leaves, or at least people do not know that this is connected in some way with the cosmos. People then describe the flower, at most thinking of a force when they want to understand the colour of a bright flower and its substances, or fertilization. People describe all those things as they would describe a person sitting down in an armchair, in exactly the same spirit; they describe it quite outwardly.

Now the essential nature of what we have to understand in the plant will not be understood at all in this way but we have to be clear that when we look at such a plant we see a wonderful secret in the roots which are lowered into the soil. And the stem with the leaves indicates another secret, as does what happens at the top with the flower.

You see, my dear friends, when we look at the root and the way it dips into the soil, this is where the plant terminates, we might say, in relation to the earth, the solid earth. But the root could not get anything from the soil if the soil were not subject first to the influence of the cosmic environment. The cosmic environment—and by that I am not just referring to the warmth and light of the sun but also to what comes from the rest of the planetary system associated with our earth—influences the earth and penetrates it a little way from the surface. And the forces which are stimulated in this way in the substances of the earth, these forces enable the root to be within the earth.

Now we can try and see where we can find these forces again. Well, these same forces that we found around the plant root are found again in the human head, but we find them there in quite a different way from how they are around the plant root in the soil. And we will not get a proper inner perception of what is happening here if we stop at what natural science can give us today. And that is what many of you refer to in your questions as the chaotic element which has been placed in your souls by the natural science of today. It is indeed necessary that we should gain living access once again also to external substances and agents, that we should gain living access to what was once called earth, water, air and fire. Because if all we ever do is talk about hydrogen, oxygen, carbon, nitrogen, sulphur, phosphorus in the way that chemistry does, these things will always have something superficial about them. You will never be able to think anything other than that you stand there as a human being and somewhere outside you there is oxygen or nitrogen. It is something quite indirect which you learn about oxygen and nitrogen through the physiology or chemistry of today. You learn through physiology that there is nitrogen in the human organism but you do not experience it there. It is important to start with those things that can be experienced. And what can be experienced must connect profoundly with the whole essence of the human being if we want to put ourselves at the service of the way that the world develops. Because that is what we do when we want to heal.

Now, one of the things that belongs with the old elements is that every person knows that they can experience them. Take warmth, for example, warmth as a quality of nature. We experience it, we become warm or feel cold. We do not experience warmth in the outward way in which we experience oxygen or nitrogen. That is the unique characteristic of the ancient way of looking at nature, that it based itself on experience which we can enter into, not which we have to stand outside of. So let us stay with the element of warmth, of fire, because that is the thing where the experience is most palpable, if I may use that paradoxical expression. We know that we experience warmth as human beings. Now the same thing which the earth, the earthy element represents for the plant root is represented for the human head by warmth. And now imagine what appears to you as the solid earth—if you have the earth here [R.S. draws]—but without the earthy element itself, the watery element, the airy element and imagine that what remains is warmth (it is quite possible to imagine that). And take the whole thing [see drawing II], you have below here and above here, and you turn it around so that you have below here and above here [I]. Then you have truly polar opposites. On the one hand you can imagine if we have below here and above here [II], and warmth has been released here as far down as the earthy element, that the plant root is in there. But

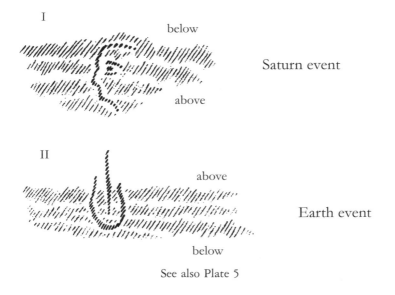

I

below

above

Saturn event

II

above

below

Earth event

See also Plate 5

when warmth is in here on its own [I], when the airy, watery and earthy elements have gone and conversely the ground is here [II], from which the warmth is gone, then, if we have the rootlike, the plantlike, here [II], we have here [I] what comes from the human head itself.

So what does that mean? My dear friends, it means this, that you can say to yourselves I look at the plant root and it is in the earthy ground. I look at the human head, it is in the warmth ground, only the ground is reversed. That is because what happens up here [I above] lies four stages back from this [II]. If we call what happens with the plant root an Earth event, then you have to call what is still happening with the head today as the result of warmth a Saturn event. In between there are Sun and Moon events. And if you now imagine the human head without all the things that later entered into it, the earthy, watery, airy elements, and you just imagine the warmth active in the head which supplies the rest of the organism with differentiated warmth, you only imagine the warmth organism present in the head, then today you have a small Saturn in the human head.

You currently have the old Saturn organization in the head. And if you understand the connection, you can say: innumerable years ago there was a development in the cosmos which anticipated all that is warmthlike in the human head. And the plant root creates an image of what happened then in the earth element today.

There you have the connection. You can see old Saturn in the warmth organization of the human head. But such an insight, if it happens in the right way, must be properly connected not just with theoretical ideas but with inner moral impulses. We have to be able to look at the human head in such a way that we say: what effect does it have on us when we look at the human head and it is there like the living, embodied memory of that ancient time of development in the cosmos, the Saturn period? Try permeating yourself with the feeling: I am a human being, on the one hand, who has reached a certain age; I think of my childhood, childhood memories arise. As a person who has grown older, I immerse myself in my childhood memories. We then have a certain inner experience before which we can stand with moral force. And now expand this feeling, this sense to the point where you say: I existed as a human being in the old Saturn period; if I understand my head correctly in the present time, it exists like a living reminder of the original time when the cosmos was created. And let me say that what is formed through the childhood memories will seem infinitely multiplied to me if we get as far as the ancient Saturn period through these childhood memories, through the living human head. All such knowledge is only of value if it is immersed directly in the moral mind, if we can feel an inner thrill because we are immersed in a feeling for the cosmos through the activity of the human being. And meditation for physicians does not mean only brooding on thoughts but meditating consists in placing such connections before our soul and through such connections inner differentiated feelings in which we can experience inner upheaval of all kinds.

You see, I might meet a person whom I have not seen for 40 years. When I meet him in his current form, I see his childhood before my soul; I see him as a child before me and that produces a certain inner upheaval. Today I look at the plant root. By looking at the plant root I develop the ability to relate the plant root to the human head and the human head takes me back to the ancient Saturn period. Meditation has to include the whole of the soul part of the human being, it has to stimulate profound inner life.

This is intended to indicate a direction in which, after the basis has been created through a kind of exoteric course, everything in the esoteric sphere must be directed towards a feeling experience of the whole cosmos in connection with the complete human being. Because just as you can gain an understanding of Saturn existence through observing the connection between the human head and the growth of the roots in the plant, the sun's existence can become clear through the connection between the human heart and the development of the stem and leaves in the plant. And conversely the development of the stem and leaves in the plant is a living memory of existence on the old Sun.

And when we rise to the flower, in which the seed is created in the plant, then we get to what is connected with the human metabolic system, the limb system. And if in this connection we look at what happens in the flower together with the human metabolic and limb system, something comes to appearance which is like a memory of the old Moon period. And if you take this inner feeling experience, my dear friends, if you really feel these connections inwardly through profound meditation, you will experience even more.

Then something very significant will happen in your soul. Then, when you turn your soul towards the plant with such deeper sentience, you will begin to have the feeling that no plant root is at rest. You will feel with regard to each plant root that it is moving. You will learn to recognize this feeling. I can only present these things in outline, I can only give an indication of an impulse on this occasion, indicate the way in which such inner experience, such knowledge of nature must be developed into wisdom. You will experience such movement of the plant roots. If you observe them in this way you will feel as if you were travelling through cosmic space with the plant root. [See Plate 5] Through this experience alone, through getting into this vehicle, as we might say, which travels through space and you travel with it at the speed of the plant root, you will experience the movement of the whole of our planetary system through space. In the plant root you experience the movement of our whole planetary system through space. And if you then go to the growth of the leaves and experience this in the way I have described, you will once again experience a kind of movement. And that is the true experience, the inner experience of the movement of the earth.

Movement of the planetary system: root.
Movement of what is connected in stem and leaf: earth movement.

What the Copernican system says about the movement of the earth around the sun is, after all, a construct. You will perceive the real movement of the earth when you study the way in which the stem and leaves are connected with one another. With the stem and leaves you are moving with the earth in concordance with the sun so that the earth looks the way in which it is described in the Copernican system. But in reality it is a much more complex movement. When you look up towards what happens in the flower—where we have the stamen and pistils—and experience that, then you will experience the movement of the moon around the earth through what happens in the flower: an experience of the movement [in what] is already separated from the earth. The whole of the planetary system including the earth is

Moon movement

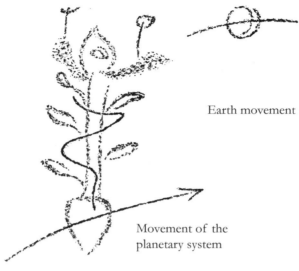

Earth movement

Movement of the
planetary system

See Plate 5

experienced in the root of the plant; the movement of the earth is experienced in the stem and leaves; the movement of the moon, i.e. those things which are already separated, is experienced in the seed production of the plant.

I tell you these things, my dear friends, so that you gain some insight into what is not taken into account at all in contemporary science because these things are not considered to be knowable or worth knowing. But they are the things which need to be known because otherwise you do not know anything at all. And I say these things also for another reason. I do not think that what someone can learn about the plants could come as a shock to them. It leaves them quite indifferent. They receive it like something to which they are indifferent. They do not go through anything. But if in the course of a second medical course, which you'll be able to attend, you learn about the planetary movements, the movement of the earth and the moon by way of the plants—something that happens in a somewhat different way also through the minerals—and by way of human beings, that will not leave you indifferent.

Indeed, my dear friends, we are faced today with the necessity of applying our way of gaining insight to things like these, and our hearts feel that the ways of gaining insight have to go along these lines. But what is offered to hearts today is something doctrinal which contains nothing of reality because people believe they have reality in what can be understood in small portions. What is the procedure in science today? It is really as follows. I always think of it as if someone were to go to Dresden to look at the *Sistine Madonna*[18] and a scientist came up to him and told him: but the *Sistine Madonna* is nothing but an outward impression. And then he would proceed to take the painting of the *Madonna* out of its frame and cut it into smaller and smaller pieces until there was a pile of atom-sized pieces. Then he would say: now you know what the *Madonna* is really like. That is not true. If we want to gain a true understanding of the *Madonna* we first of all have to understand religious intentions through what religion can offer us. Then we have to see what was put into the *Madonna* through the spirituality of Raphael,[19] and many other things. But that would be the next step. And in this way we have to attempt to understand the intentions of the gods, the divine spiritual beings who are behind what is physical. That will have to be explained in the second course. And only in this way is it possible to bring people close to reality.

So if you take what I have spoken about now as a suggestion, you will be able to understand the two meditations which will awaken powers of gaining medical insight in you in the way I spoke them yesterday. And you can do this meditation such that at first you simply immerse yourself in the external appearance of fire, of warming fire, and that you learn to comprehend with heartfelt seriousness that this outer appearance of fire is external maya, appearance, illusion. But behind the fire something quite different is at work, behind the fire there is active will, active will. [See Plate 5]

You might well ask, how do I recognize that there is active will behind fire. It has always been the case in esoteric schools and what comes from these schools that an appeal is made to the pupils themselves. If you simply allow what I have told you today to enter your mind, you will begin to understand inwardly that there is active will wherever there is fire, just as you begin to understand that there is spirit and soul when you see the shape of a human face, a human form. Wherever you find fire, in the smallest match, there is active will. From the beginning there is active will where there is fire. And in order to be able to penetrate the other substances of nature you have to develop this to a stage in which a burning match is not just the external appearance to you as which it is described today but that you perceive it as active will. Because if you can transform your mind in this way, truly transform it, then you will find that your soul begins to feel in quite a different way; it will adopt a completely different attitude to your surroundings. Then you will not just experience things as you do when you live in reality. You will feel yourself connected in your own active will with what is fire. You will immerse yourself from your own human being in the world and will truly be able to experience fire in a much finer way than previously because the affinity with your own will appears. You will experience this affinity wherever fire appears. You must learn: I am in this fire because it is active will, it is part of me like my finger is.

You will only experience air in your being if you experience it as courage. Everywhere where wind occurs, wind blowing in nature, you will feel it in your own soul as courage. So what you see in external nature as air is courage. Courage is air. You should experience that in your soul.

Water is the external appearance of sentience. Where sentience occurs, something is at work inwardly which appears outwardly as water. Water is sentience.

And where there is earth, the solid earth, such firmness is the same thing as the thought. After all, life freezes in the thought.

If you can grasp these four thoughts in meditation, if you can learn to think that fire is active will, if you can take the external appearance of fire as a revelation of the active will, if you can approach fire in such a way that you see active will in it in the same way that you see spirit and soul in the human form, if you can sense that the outer form of fire is maya, if in the blowing wind, in the clouds you can sense that these are the phenomena that reveal courage, if you can see water as sentience coming to appearance everywhere in the world, if you can see something in earth everywhere that is equal to your thoughts, then you will find the path which will enable you to recognize in yourselves what we can discuss in these eight days: that the organic process occurring in you as earth formation starting from the head and extending downwards, that this organic process is continuous earth formation, bringing together something of substance in earth formation, and that this is the essence of the thought.

If you move to the essence of respiration, if you feel how in respiration the aeriform part of the human being circulates, then you will recognize in the aeriform, in the action of the aeriform in human beings everything that is activity in human beings, that leads human beings into the external world to assert themselves in the external world. And you will seek to learn from a variety of phenomena in nature what happens with air in human beings themselves.

And you will recognize how sentience, sentience working centrifugally and centripetally, lives in everything connected with the watery element, the water or fluid organism in human beings with its inner flexibility. You will recognize what is movement in the air through a semicircular movement, a movement from the top downwards. You will recognize that what lives in the fluid is centripetal and centrifugal movement in human beings, always seeking to maintain an equilibrium. You will learn to find the transition to what happens with the elements inside human beings through observing what nature does externally. But the prerequisite is that we do not stop at ordinary observation, because all normal observation turns us into earth ourselves, dries us out and makes us fixed so that we lose all flexibility.

There is a lot in what I have told you in outline today; I have left out all kinds of intermediary stages. But I cannot tell you every detail, that would take too long. I can only point you in the right direction. You can see from this that there will have to be a change in the way in which courses are organized today. So it is up to you to see that the things which I have pointed out here can truly bear fruit in you. To this end it is necessary that you answer a large part of the questions you have asked with a heavy heart, and which I read with a heavy heart because they indicate in such a profound way what our time requires today—that you answer some of these questions by remaining in permanent contact with the Goetheanum. In that way you will experience a constant fertilization of your medical studies wherever you may undertake them. That of course requires that you truly have the feeling that you must work seriously at your studies. Some serious work has to be done. And you must have another feeling which has to come very sincerely and honestly from within yourselves. You must decide, or not, that in the coming period medical studies must be fertilized from Dornach. And medical studies will be fertilized from Dornach in the way that is required so that the path is chosen in medicine which must be followed.

Then another issue will be the question of karma. Because of course anyone who wants to heal must have an intimate relationship with karma in the world. Well, I will speak further about that in the next few sessions. You cannot heal by going against karma. You can only heal as is required by karma. But karma is not something where you can superficially say: if someone is ill, let them stay ill, that is their karma; and if they become healthy again that is karma too. We must not make those kinds of judgement. The question as to how karma in particular works in human life requires thorough cosmic deepening. These things will be done from Dornach for those who seek them.

I have already said that these impulses will be given in future from truly esoteric sources, because it is necessary for those things to be taken into account which simply exist as realities and which were strongly envisaged at the Christmas Conference when the General Anthroposophical Society was founded. With regard to the field of medicine they are the following. In a much deeper sense than I already mentioned yesterday I am not worried about whether others copy the medicines if only people in future properly understand in a much deeper sense that esoteric medical studies should be undertaken in connection with Dornach. That requires that medical studies should be undertaken in future in the same way as the other branches of spiritual life in Dornach. You see, it has always been the case in the life of the Anthroposophical Society that all the personalities who wanted to become esotericists did not observe the conditions of esoteric life, simply the inner conditions of esoteric life, thoroughly enough. And so within the anthroposophical movement we have over the years been able to achieve what is required really only in two areas, namely in the field of general anthroposophy and the field of eurythmy and the art of speech. But what has developed in these fields as inner activity, as independent inner activity, must truly develop in all the sections which are now to be set up. And that means submitting in full trust to the conditions which are being established from herein. These conditions include that in the first instance I will have to do all the things which need to be done in the medical field together with Dr Wegman, who has prepared herself for the medical field throughout the course of the anthroposophical movement and is now so much part of this whole medical stream that she must lead it together with me. So only those will be able to find their way with guidance from Dornach who follow Dr Wegman in trust. That is why we will have to establish in the coming period that those who wish to remain in constant contact with the Section for the Revitalization of Medicine should turn to Dr Wegman with their concerns in full and absolute trust in a form which we can still discuss further. We will answer the corresponding questions periodically, perhaps monthly, in a newsletter for those who at the end of this course have thereby, as it were, become students at the Dornach Goetheanum. That is how it will be in this and in the other sections. These newsletters will answer the questions put by individuals and all those involved in the section concerned will receive the answers. But this will not work without inner trust. That creates a real relationship and all your human and medical requirements will be met in the immediate future. It will initially be set up in this way, and then we can proceed to set up further facilities in order to create a connection in this way.

The great error which occurred in our esoteric life until now was that people thought in great arrogance that they should all receive their esoteric exercises only from me. Everyone wants to deal with me and with no one else. That is what has caused our esoteric work to fail so far! But the inner occult foundations dictate that what lives in the esoteric sources must be passed on through the appropriate people. It is part of esotericism that the personalities determined by destiny to do so must pass on this esoteric material. That was rejected because people were insufficiently modest in their demands. But if nothing changes we will not, of course, get any further in the newly founded Anthroposophical Society either. It has to happen.

Thus far what I have initially presented in outline. I will go on to explain in greater detail how the esoteric work has to continue. I just wanted to present this to you and will continue with our esoteric observations tomorrow. Then I truly intend to answer the majority of your questions which all amount to this one thing: how do I find a path of schooling which comes from Dornach? You can find it, but you must have trust. That does not mean a blind belief in authority but meaningfully building on a foundation, an inner foundation, accepting the conditions which have been created by destiny. That's it for today, then. We will continue tomorrow. Don't worry, I will deal with individual questions to the extent that they require to be answered in this way. [See Plate 5]

Fire	active will
Air	courage
Water	sensibility
Earth	thoughts

LECTURE 6

My dear friends,
For reasons I do not want to discuss right now, I will hold the more esoterically oriented session I intended for today at the end of the course.

Today I want to talk to you about something else. If we recall what we said yesterday, we might be a bit surprised that we should see thought forms behind the appearance of what is solid and earthy, that we should see courage behind the aeriform if we want to get close to the realities. Now it is also of what I would like to call a certain medical and historical importance that we pay attention in the right way to how thoughts should be combined with what is solid and earthy, what is contoured in our perception, because that is also how we directly realize something else. Namely that the thought should not be combined with what is fluid, with the fluid and other circulation in the human organism, that we should not see thoughts as the force behind it or behind the aeriform and warmthlike. We have seen how we should think of the aeriform and warmthlike in the cosmos. But everything is present in turn in human beings in a special form. In human beings this form is such that only those things which have contours, which—even if they are what we might roughly or superficially call soft—still have the character of something solid through their contoured nature, can enter thoughts, and that we must be clear that behind the fluid of which we spoke we have to see something connected with sentience if we want to understand the spiritual behind the ordinary physical plane.

Thus what is related to sentience in the human organism must be seen separately because ordinarily the subjective sensations which human beings have through their soul and physical constitution are at work when we talk about sentience. But in human beings sentience is not just what we directly experience. In human beings sentience has an anabolic effect; and because the fluid body as a form of a general cosmic fluidity by its nature already contains what is connected with sentience, we must be clear that what is at work in the fluid body—these etheric impulses—must also be understood with our powers of insight. But we cannot understand it with our cognition in the way we understand things which are outside the human organism because in the human organism everything which we encounter as substances or processes changes in relation to the human being's environment. And thus we have to understand that at the point where the fluid organism starts— where we are dealing with a part of the human organization which is in fluid circulation, even if vascular organs or other things form part of the structure of such circulation—all the cognitive forces which apply to what is outside the human being in the physical world are no longer of use for understanding these matters.

That is why, you see, it has come about that medicine has lost sight of the fluid human being as the last component of the human organization. It would be true to say that until the mid-1840s medicine at least still had some idea of the fluid human being. There was reference to the humours, to the fluid circulation, to mixing and separation of fluids. Not only was there cellular physiology and pathology at the time, but there was a real understanding of the mixing and separation of fluids. Of course it was all traditional knowledge in the nineteenth century. But this tradition went back to a period lying before the sixteenth and fifteenth centuries, in which there was not just such a tradition but real knowledge, knowledge of the type we need to strive for, recover again in anthroposophy today through Imagination. That previous time had an imaginative character but they were instinctive imaginations. And it was known that the human organism could not simply be understood through mere sensory perception and reflection. Thoughts and sensory perceptions only take us to the firmly contoured parts of the organism; everything that involves the fluid circulation in the fluid human being must be understood through imagination. It is therefore no great surprise that this perception of the fluid human being has been lost because the old instinctive imagination has been lost. Such perception will only return when imaginations are achieved in full consciousness. Let us try to bring together what we have spoken about and what is in prospect for cognition. [See Plate 6]

You see, as the skeleton is built up out of the totality of the human organism, as human beings crystallize into the skeleton—that is not a good way of putting it but you will understand what I mean—cosmic thoughts are at work on them. And the strictly contoured organs are only strictly contoured because they are subject to the same forces—we will learn about their real forces directly—to which the development of the bones is subject. So we can say that only the bone structure has thought quality in a physical sense and the other organs with solid contours grow out of the etheric in a way that has thought quality. But because they have solid contours they are thought structures and what you have in physiology and pathology today in terms of the form of the human organism is a principle that has thought quality. But that is only one component of the human organism and it must drop out of the human organization if we do not rise to the imaginative level. Imagination then leads us up to the fluid human being and the way that the muscles are formed out of fluid and the human being shoots into the muscle. This curious assemblage of the apparently firm muscle, which only appears solid, and the blood—at that point we already move from the bonelike to the blood where we have to use the imagination to understand the human being. [See Plate 6] So we can say that the thought, which is naturally supported by sensory perception, only reaches as far as the skeletal system and anything else we say about the human being through thinking other than about the skeletal system is nonsense. We have to rise from the thinking to Imagination. And when we rise to the Imagination we come to the fluid human being and how the fluid human being really shoots into the muscular system. We can only understand the nature of muscles through Imagination. Why?

Well, you see, if you use thoughts you also have to apply the laws which are subject to the thinking, that is, mechanical laws. You have to use statics and dynamics. But you can only do that with the skeletal system. But try using statics and dynamics with the muscular system, try to calculate on the basis of statics why you are able to crack a cherry stone with your teeth, or indeed a peach stone. Try to calculate that. Try setting up an experiment to measure how much weight pressure is required for that—simply by placing a weight on a cherry stone—to crack such a cherry stone. You can bite it in two, perhaps not all of us, but there are people who can bite a peach stone in two. Calculate whether according to mechanical laws a muscle can manage to bite a cherry stone in two. With the material provided by thoughts you will never get close to the muscular system. You cannot do that. Mechanics become a nonsense as soon as we are dealing with muscles and we must be able to make the transition to a kind of knowledge which can leave the mechanical laws to one side, that is, which has an understanding of the muscles through Imagination where ordinary gravity does not come in. Because as soon as you are dealing with fluids you are dealing with buoyancy and you do the things you do with your etheric body, not through weight but through those things which largely overcome weight. So on that basis alone you will understand that as soon as we approach the muscular system we have to use a quite different cognitive method, that is, Imagination, so that we can say—only in a representative way, there are transitional stages in every instance—that the muscular system is understood with Imagination.

And no one will understand the muscular system who fails to see it in a sense as an image which has not arisen in the same way as the skeletal system but which has formed in a sense through the coagulation of the blood. This is of course as much an inept expression as when I say crystallized into the skeletal system, but it is comparatively correct. So just think when you have a bone, say the ulna or radius or the upper arm, and you apply the lever rule to it. Well, the bones are quite happy to have that done to them. But consider—while you can understand quite well what happens with the radius or the upper arm through leverage and other mechanical laws—whether you can also understand what is happening in any given muscle. There the images have to take on a soft structure, have to be transformed. That is precisely the nature of an imagination that it can yield everywhere and that it comprises those things which acquire their substance through metamorphosis. The muscle possesses that, the muscle lives in its metamorphosis. Bones patiently subject themselves to the laws of mechanics, the muscles do not. They are just as flexible as the metamorphosing images—images, not thoughts—which we have in the imagination to follow them in our inner flexibility. So you see, with the solid, earthy human being we are in the skeletal system. With the muscular system we are in the fluid human being.

If we now rise from Imagination to Inspiration, we get to the aeriform human being, those things in the human being which are aeriform. And in coming close to Inspiration we are getting to a way of comprehension that is very similar to hearing musical tones, harmonies, melodies, very similar to musical listening. Inspiration no longer has anything to do with anything conceptual but with something which is musical even in the way we perceive it. Something musical does not always need to be heard; it can also be sensed if it is spiritual. And all Inspiration fundamentally has something musical. Now we have the peculiar thing here that the form of the human internal organs—those organs which take care of the development of our organization throughout life in respiration, nutrition and so on, that is, the organs underlying all those things—those organic forms cannot be explained by any mechanical laws. But they cannot be explained imaginatively either. It is simply absurd, nonsense if we wanted to explain the form of the lungs or the liver simply in terms of their structure, how the cells are organized, or by weight. Just take a look and see whether anyone has succeeded yet in explaining the form of the lung or liver as form. No one has managed to do that. Because these organs, which take care of developing life during our time on earth, exist at a very early primordial stage even if in a very strongly metamorphosed form. They all have their origin in the formative aeriform forces.

Today's scientifically inclined person says that air is made up of oxygen, nitrogen, a number of other things, and it is a more or less regular substance which is only differentiated through inner mechanical movement which manifests itself in the form of wind. But the kind of air that the physicist describes today does not exist. There is only the concrete air that surrounds our earth. But, my dear friends, the air that surrounds our earth is permeated everywhere with formative forces. We inhale these formative forces with the physical substance of the air. Once our organs are complete, when we have a finished lung, then it happens that the formative forces which we inhale with the substance of the air coincide, as it were, with the form of the lung so that they no longer have any great importance once we are born except for growth. But during the embryonic period, during the physical separation from the external air, that is when the formative forces of the air are at work initially through the maternal body, they build up the lung like all human organs are built up from them with the exception of the muscles and the bones. All the internal organs which preserve developing life are built up from the formative forces of the air. What happens there can be compared, albeit in a crude comparison, with the creation of Chladni figures.[20] These are plates which are lightly covered in fine particles and attached to a single point. They are bowed with a violin bow in a particular way creating specific forms depending on how they are bowed. The figures are created out of the formative forces which are called up in the air. In the same way the internal organs of the human being are formed out of the general formative forces of the air. The lung is indeed formed from the respiratory forces, but the other organs also. The only difference is that the other organs are formed more or less indirectly whereas the lung is formed directly. But the way in which the human organs are formed out of the formative oscillations of the air can only be understood through Inspiration. What forms out of the air is similar to music in the way it is perceived, just as the sound patterns also have a musical foundation.

There is so much in physiology today that is fundamentally wrong that one is sometimes embarrassed to say the right thing when it is so grotesquely different from what people say. When human beings hear, all their organs vibrate along with the vibration of the air, not just the inner hearing organs. The whole human being vibrates along, if only quietly, and therefore the ear is not an organ of hearing because it vibrates but because it brings what is present in the rest of the organism to consciousness in the way it is inwardly organized. It is a big but subtle difference if we say human beings hear through their ears or human beings use their ears to bring to consciousness what they hear. Because human beings are built up out of sound, even if that does not mean the sounds we hear, so that we have to say that Inspiration grasps the human internal organs. [See Plate 6] The organization of the human internal organs, the aeriform human being, must be understood through Inspiration. You see, it is no real surprise that a real understanding of the human organs was lost even in ancient times because Inspiration was lost, and because Inspiration is the only way to understand the internal organs. Otherwise all we can do is look at their shape in a corpse but we will not understand them.

So you can see that really the whole human organism exists in the background of the physical world. When we talk in the way I have done in my book *Knowledge of the Higher Worlds. How is it Achieved?*[21] people always imagine that here we have the physical world and behind it we have the spiritual world in stages. We get into the closest spiritual world through Imagination, into the one after that through Inspiration and into a further one through Intuition. But people simply do not think that of all the things which make up the human being only the skeletal system is built up by the elemental spirits while the muscular system is built up by the spiritual beings of a higher hierarchy. That has to be recognized now. We must be able to go to these beings through Imagination if we want to understand the muscular system. Equally we have to go to even higher spiritual beings through Inspiration if we want to understand the internal organs. By putting your skeleton upright you only look as if you were adapted to the shapes. But in its inner development the skeleton can only be investigated by means of Inspiration.

You have to see what I want to say in the following way. Today's researchers think about or study a plant by analysing what they can see, the substance presented to them, using the methods commonly applied today. But that is not the plant. The plant is structured in the way that I explained yesterday. It is built out of the cosmos and only the root has a physical construction. The whole form of the plant is spiritual reality, supersensory reality; but the supersensory has been filled with matter. And anyone who simply investigates this physical matter in the plant is like a person who has a text before him where the ink is still wet, covers it with blotting sand and then thinks that the blotting sand represents the essence of the text. When they study a plant today, people are acting like someone who has a text before him and covers it with blotting sand because the ink is still wet. Then he scrapes off the sand and says, I will study the sand to see what is written in the text. That, broadly, is how people attempt to explain a plant whereas in reality it is a spiritual being which is only filled within its space with physical substance. In the same way the human organ systems are only filled with physical substance. In reality only the skeletal system is physical, the muscular system is etheric and the organ system is astral. [See Plate 6]

And if we rise to true Intuition we reach the warmth human being, the organization which is a space filled with inwardly differentiated warmth. Now I said that we truly experience ourselves in warmth, that we do not experience it like carbon or nitrogen, but warmth just is; it is inside us and we are in it when we experience it. It is precisely the thing which we experience most intensively. That is why people today cannot deny that they experience warmth whereas they have no idea that they experience air, water and earth. They have no idea because they have grown out of that. But the experience of warmth is the direct application of Intuition to the human organism. We simply have to experience warmth not in a wholesale way, as we do in ordinary life, but in the way it is finely differentiated in the forms of the organs themselves. If we are able to observe the warmth organism throughout the organism by means of Intuition, this cognitive method will lead us to an understanding not of the internal organs but of the activity of the internal organs. All the activity of the internal organs must be grasped through an understanding of the way that the warmth ether is organized. Anything else is not really suitable for achieving an understanding of the activity of the organs.

A perception, an intuitive perception of the activity of the warmth ether, that is, of the warmth human being—that is what must be understood through Intuition. In other words, it is not sufficient simply to think that here we have the physical world and then we acquire Imagination, Inspiration and Intuition to enter other worlds. The other worlds are here. The etheric world is here in that human beings have a muscular system, the astral world is here in that human beings have a system of organs, and the world of Devachan, the spiritual world is here in that we have the warmth human being. The spiritual is constantly among us. It is here. After all, the human being is a spirit, but this spirit is filled with physical substance. That is why we abandon ourselves to the illusion that human beings are only physical beings. Human beings are even spirit as such, reaching up through the warmth organization into the highest world that can be reached. That is why it is so amusing to see eight or ten spiritualists sitting around a table calling on spirits which are much, much lower than the eight or ten people who are sitting around the table and do not know that they, too, are spirit. That, my dear friends, is something of which we must be deeply aware—then we can begin to move to a higher level. [See Plate 6]

Thought	Skeletal system	= solid, earthy h[uman being]
Imagination	Muscular system	= fluid watery h[uman being]
Inspiration	Internal organs	= airy[form] h[uman being]
Intuition	Activity of the internal organs	= warmth human being

You see, once we have grasped through Intuition the activity, this wonderful activity within the whole human organization from one organ to the next, all the things that take place in the warmth ether, we find that there are two types of warmth. The warmth ether is a very special element. If there is any process which produces a change in the warmth ether there is always a reaction. By their nature warmth currents always flow counter to one another—action and reaction. The warmth ether is differentiated within itself. There is always a cruder etheric substance which is opposed by a finer etheric substance. But only that makes it possible for phenomena to appear which we can illustrate in the first instance with a crude image. Imagine that you were in a heated room which is nice and warm; it is pleasant. You heat it up to such an extent that you can no longer stand it. That is not just a physical state, it is also a mental state. The one warmth, the finer warmth, is experienced particularly by the soul. We always experience warmth in two ways: the warmth we experience in the soul and the warmth in which we live, which is outside our soul; the warmth which is in our warmth organism and the warmth which is outside. We can say that there is physical warmth and mental warmth.

But if we take the internal organs, the aeriform human being which is comprehended through Inspiration, we have the airy element in its main form to begin with. But this airy form has light working within it—in a different way from the way that the finer warmth is at work in warmth itself. So we can say that for intuition warmth becomes comprehensible in warmth; warmth remains warmth in that it is differentiated within its own element. But that is not the case with air. The real air is not the fantastical air of the physicists, which surrounds our earth like a skin; that does not exist. The real air cannot be thought without a light state—and darkness is also a light state—so that air and light represent an associated differentiation; light is an organizing component in the whole air organism. Now we progress even further into the soul entity. There is not just external light but also metamorphosed inner light which penetrates the whole human being, which lives in him or her. Light lives in human beings through the air.

And, equally, the chemical metabolism lives in you through water, through the fluid element. That is where the chemical forces reside. Water imagined as physical water, that is, the water of the physicists, is fantasy. At the moment that water appears anywhere in an organizing capacity; it always appears with the chemical metabolism. Imagining the fluid element in human beings without the chemical metabolism is like imagining a human organism without the head. We can even draw it, eliminate everything of a soul nature, but it is no longer a reality. Your body can no longer live if you cut the head off—it no longer remains an organism. Equally the fluid element in the human being is not what physicists describe fantastically as water, but just as the human organism forms an integrated whole with the head so the chemical metabolism is tied to the fluid everywhere.

And the solid or earthy part of the human organism is only present in the nascent state just as water is only present in the latter state in human beings. It is transformed immediately. The earthy element is only present in human beings when it is tied simultaneously to life. [See also Plate 7]

Earth	Life
Water	Chemical metabolism
Air	Light
Warmth	In warmth
Phys[ical] [body]	eth[eric] body

And now, you see, if you draw a—vertical—line here you have the physical body here and the associated etheric body here. But they are a single whole, are only two sides of the same coin we might say. You have the etheric states of warmth, light, the chemical metabolism and life and the physical states of warmth, air, water and earth. Well, if we were to describe the etheric states in abstract, we would first look at the warmth ether as the lowest ether in the context of fluidity, solidity and so on. The next highest ether would be the life ether. But when we describe the human being we have to proceed in such a way that Intuition gets to know the warmth human being, the inner activity of the organs. In climbing down to the most crude level, from the warmth to the earthy element, we climb up in the etheric body from warmth to life. What does that mean? Just consider: human beings actually reverse the human qualities. They only apply the warmth ether to the warmth organization, the light ether to the air organism, the chemical ether to the fluid organization, the life ether to the solid organization. If you really understand something like that you cannot think as people normally think. If you want to stop and only think like people normally think, you can really only understand the skeletal human being, the earth human being. You need to progress from normal thinking to such an understanding of the world which truly inwardly takes hold of you, as I said before.

And so you see, my dear friends, that is why in the end there is something special about medical knowledge. In the ancient mysteries, where certain insights existed regarding the treatment of human beings, medical knowledge was an outstanding part of the mysteries. The physicians were trained in the mysteries and were not just physicians but also wise people who took care of the religious cults. In that context it was relatively natural that the physician kept his knowledge, as indeed all mystery knowledge, secret in a certain sense. Because you see, if we want to know something we have to clothe that knowledge in thoughts, otherwise we would drift in indeterminacy. The pictorial knowledge in Imagination, the knowledge which is spiritually heard and intuitively seen must be clothed in thoughts. Now people say about these thoughts, like about the thoughts of modern anthroposophy, that they are not expressed very well. It was clear to people that medical knowledge had to be transformed into thoughts. By transforming medical knowledge into thoughts something of its effectiveness is removed if it is therapeutic knowledge. I am touching on something here which is connected with very profound things. It cannot be denied that knowledge about medicines removes the strength of those medicines in a certain sense; and it is necessary for a physician who wishes to be taken seriously to forgo in his own case to a greater or lesser extent the efficacy of the medicines which he uses for his patients and to observe different ways of healing for himself. Please consider what this sentence implies and you will realize that, in a much deeper sense than what has been said hitherto, the physician must develop a personal disposition of wanting to give assistance. He really in his own case has to forgo the healing powers with regard to those things which he uses for his patients. If we crudely ascribe the efficacy of medicines to chemical forces, if we believe that medicines work like the steam in a locomotive, then we are not subject to such spiritual laws. But if we see how human beings extend into the spiritual realm we will not doubt for a minute that spiritual laws underlie the foundations of the different medicines specially for human beings. If it is grasped in its true essence, medicine is to the highest degree the most wonderful way to educate ourselves to be selfless. That is why in a certain sense it is a gross, a colossally gross misunderstanding if people keep demanding today that all therapy should be taught in the same way as mechanics or similar things. After all, mechanics can be applied to the individual human being but also to the whole of humanity. With a physician everything is individual and if he or she has a real, in-depth knowledge of a medicine there is a high degree of necessity for that physician to forgo using the medicine in his or her own treatment. That is the great education in selflessness. I will still speak about how physicians can nevertheless help themselves. But the things which underlie such facts should take root in your hearts. If you take the things seriously which I have just spoken about today, then it will happen simply as a result of universal laws that altruism and not egoism will be introduced into medicine. That is already inherent in the basic attitude. And altruism, selflessness, is the basic element of medicine. Medical ethics is not just something artificial but a consequence of heaven's very own laws, laws which have been formed by the cosmos in order to create medicines on the basis of those laws.

The more such information induces a serious mood, the more it will be able to contribute to capturing the real essence of the medicines as such.

LECTURE 7

My dear friends,
We will use the first part of today's session to answer those questions which were not included in the general question which I have already discussed and which will still be discussed further. And we will then continue today with the discussion from yesterday in order then to lead to an esoteric conclusion tomorrow.

Most of the questions actually fit into what I want to say to you in general. There are only a few questions that require a specific answer and we will deal with them in no particular order.

Question: Are there specific exercises to strengthen the so-called forces of magnetic healing in us and what are those exercises?

Well, that of course requires that we say a few words about magnetic healing forces as such. Magnetic healing forces are forces which essentially act between the etheric body of one person and the etheric body of another person. You then have to imagine that the effect of so-called magnetic healing is based on the following. Let us assume someone has a strong personality, that is, he can strongly develop his will and can be given instructions based on particular circumstances. Let us say, for example, that I tell him if he suffers from a particular illness he should think of the sun at eleven o'clock each morning and imagine that the sun first warms his head, that then the warmth of the head is transferred to the upper arms, the lower arms and hands, so that he reinforces his real strength in this way; then, once he has reinforced his real strength, he should try to picture very clearly what he experiences of his illness in order to get rid of it through his strength of will. This procedure, as I have described it, can—I say can because it does not happen necessarily, there is always a slight problem with these things—indeed help with the illness if there is no particular organ damage; organ damage can, of course, extend to all four members of the elementary body, the solid, fluid, gaseous and warmth one. Then the following has happened: the person concerned has been stimulated in his astral body through the instruction I have given him. My instruction which he carried out, imagining the sun, the warmth in his head and so on, this instruction which he carried out and which strengthened his will, had an effect on the astral body. The astral body worked on his etheric body and the etheric body in turn had a healing effect on his physical body to balance, to paralyse damage it has suffered which was not of a deeper organic nature. We cannot say that such cures only occur in what today's medicine calls functional disorders as opposed to organic disorders in which there is an actual disorder of the organs. Such differentiation is very imprecise. We cannot say where functional disorders stop and the organic ones start. Functional disorders are always also minor organic disorders which only cannot be shown with today's crude physiological and pathological resources. As you can see, in such a case we do not use the forces of magnetic healing but appeal to the patient to heal himself. That really is the better option under all circumstances, when it is available. As a result the will of the patient is strengthened and enhanced as we cure him.

We can also do the following: we can influence our own etheric body with our astral body, without the other person exerting his will, in such a way that our etheric body acts on the etheric body of the patient in the same way as the astral body acted previously. That is what magnetic healing consists of; the practitioner of magnetic healing does that unconsciously, he influences his own etheric body from his astral body. He can guide the forces he develops by that means instinctively to where they strengthen the forces of the patient by transferring his forces to the patient. We must be clear when we are talking about healing that the practitioner must use whatever can lead to a cure. If we are dealing with a patient who is simply weak, of whom much cannot be asked with regard to his will, we can also, on occasion, use the forces of magnetic healing. But I want to make it expressly clear that magnetic healing forces are in fact something quite problematical which cannot be used in the same way from one case to the next. For this instinctive ability which I have described, where we activate our own astral body in order to influence the etheric body by that means, this instinctive ability is an individual one. There are people who have it strongly and there are people in whom it is only weak and then there are those who do not have it at all; so there are indeed practitioners of magnetic healing who are capable of it through their aptitude. But the key thing is that, as a rule, this ability exists only for a limited time. Practitioners with this ability have such magnetism, as it is called. When they start to use it, it is very effective. But after a while it begins to weaken and that is when quackery begins in such practitioners because their ability has receded but they still act as if they continued to have it. That is the worrying thing every time magnetic healing becomes an occupation. Basically this kind of healing cannot become an occupation. That is what can be said about it. The magnetic healing process is only effective—if we have the ability at all— if it is practised with truly genuine and honest empathy with the patient which goes right down into our own organism. If you practise magnetic healing out of true love for the patient you cannot do it as an occupation. If true love is present then it will lead to something positive under all circumstances unless damage occurs from somewhere else. But in such an event it can only be practised occasionally when, driven by karma, we encounter a person whom we can help in a loving way. Then the outward sign can be the laying on of hands or stroking and what acts is that the astral body transfers its power to the etheric body which acts on the etheric body of the other person.

We should also explain from a different perspective what happens in such a case. Healing always comes from the astral body, either our own astral body or ultimately the astral body of the practitioner of magnetic healing. The reverse process underlies treatment with medicines. When you treat someone with medicines you are not doing anything other than putting substances into the physical body which then act in such a way—partly corresponding to inner forces, partly to the rhythm of the physical body—that the etheric body of the patient is influenced. Healing always comes from the etheric body. On the one hand you influence the etheric body from the astral body, that is, psychic healing which includes magnetic healing; the latter, however, has something problematical or only something that I might call humanitarian, something social, something that includes the relationship between one person and another. Or alternatively you have rational therapy which is based on medicinal intervention. It moves from the physical body down into the etheric body. But healing always has to come from the etheric body. It is complete wishful thinking that the physical body, if it becomes ill, can bring about any sort of healing. The physical body has the causes of illness within itself; the causes of healing must always come from the etheric body.

Question: What is the relationship between the heart and the female uterus and its position and soul experiences, pain and joy?

There are directly associated experiences. Firstly, the heart and uterus are two associated organs even if they are not in direct contact, belonging together like the sun and the moon. Sun and moon are associated in such a way that they both throw the same light on something. In the one instance the sun throws light directly on some-

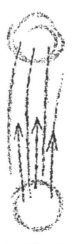

See Plate 8

thing, in the other by way of the moon from whence it is reflected. The organ of the heart has immediate, direct impulses for the human organism. It is the organ of perception for the blood circulation which takes place in the normal human organism. The female uterus is designed to be the organ of perception of the circulation which arises after fertilization. That is what it is there for; just like the moon reflects the sunlight, so the female uterus reflects the perception of the heart in the blood circulation. It reflects it back. They always belong together like the sun and moon in that their perceptions behave like direct and reflected effects. When human beings are here, they need heart forces; when they are being created they need reflected heart forces—these come from the female uterus.

Now these organs, heart and uterus, together with some others—the lung takes it more towards the etheric and physical body—are nothing other than the physical manifestation of the soul element in human beings when looked at from a spiritual perspective. Let me put it like this. Think that you develop imaginative perception. If, in looking at a human being, you develop imaginative knowledge, you really do get an image of sun and moon when you look at heart and uterus. That is indeed the corresponding spiritual element which a person experiences in their soul so that there is a real correspondence between the things which happen in the heart and the uterus; they do, however, happen in the semi-consciousness of the soul element because normally the latter is influenced by thoughts. Thus a delicate process is hidden: the intimate connection between the heart and the uterus. But anyone who has a modicum of observation can see how much depends on that, how half unconsciously or, rather, half consciously the heart activity must develop under the influence of the physical environment. Someone who lives their life in such a way that they constantly experience a shock, through their work maybe, has a precise subconscious likeness in their soul of the heart activity that arises as a result; and that is reflected in the uterus. We can see how that happens, how it is transferred to the constitution of the embryo.

Now we have a question which is difficult to answer because it must either be answered superficially, that is, simply by providing some information, or we have to deal with it thoroughly.

Question: How does wearing pearls and precious stones affect the individual organs?

It does have an effect, but it works in such a way that we can really only judge its action if we look into the spiritual worlds, and we can only judge its action individually. We can easily say, for example, that sapphire acts on a particular temperament, on a choleric, but really only in individual cases. There are effects but if we wanted to answer the question fully we would have to deal with deeper things which is not possible today.

I can only answer this question:

How can we gain insight into karma with regard to individual illnesses?

on the basis of what I said in the session. Some things will have become clear from what I said, some things will still emerge from what I still have to say.

Now we have a number of questions here and we also have the general questions which can be answered with the esoteric remarks I made. But now we have here:

Question: Are there valid parallel relationships between the degree and length of post-mortem decomposition processes and the destiny of the associated individual in the spiritual world?

There are really no relationships of any importance which would concern us human beings. It is, however, the case that the decomposition process is not just the physical process which it is normally considered to be in chemistry. Something deeply spiritual is, indeed, linked with it. People had a feeling for that in the old instinctive knowledge. We say that the innermost core of a matter is its essence and in decomposition we have a movement towards the essence [Translator's note: The German term used here by Steiner for decomposition is *verwesen*, which is made up of the elements 'ver' and 'wesen'. *Wesen* in German means 'essence' or 'being'. Steiner here points out that the prefix 'ver' indicates movement towards something so in *verwesen* that would be movement towards the essence.] Humans are not closed off beings. Spiritual beings are at work in them. We have certain beings in the physical, etheric and astral body; we are only free in the I-organization. These beings associated with the physical, etheric and astral body are associated with what happens with the physical body after death. The question of decomposition or cremation is intimately connected with this. But all these things are intimately connected with human karma. We can only say that for the human being as such—for the individual human being—the question is not necessarily of any great significance.

Question: Is there a certain period after death following which a post-mortem examination influences the destiny of the deceased?

It is completely without influence on the destiny of the deceased.

Most of the questions have been answered in the general lectures. Oh yes, there is still one question which is of a certain importance.

Question: My question is, are the healing abilities of physicians purely personal in nature or are they dependent on a communal situation? Not a communal situation between the physician and patient, that is, but between communities of physicians. Is it possible that powers flow to the individual physician through such communities which perhaps one might not be able to have at all by oneself, as is also the case in the community of priests?

That is indeed the case, only it is the case in every human community. It is the case in every human community that powers flow to the human being from out of the community; but the community has to be a real community. It has to be felt, perceived, experienced. And what I have described to you and will describe even more clearly tomorrow is of such a nature that it can form a community among you together with us here, even if it initially can only be a community by correspondence. It should unite you in such a way that when you are alone you will feel that powers will flow to you through such community not just by intellectual but also by spiritual means.

A small group[22] focused on this question:

Training a physician's eye. Are iris diagnosis, graphology, palmistry of value?

Well, in an ideal situation someone who can observe these connections could see an extraordinary amount about the overall state of a person from a small piece of fingernail you cut off for example. That is quite possible. Just as you can see an exceptional amount from a human hair. You only have to consider how individual, how different a hair, for example, can be with regard to a person. You only have to consider how broadly, I might say, people are differentiated with regard to their hair. There are blond people among you and people with black hair. Where does that come from? In those people with black hair the blackness comes from an iron process which takes place in the hair. Those who are blond have their blondness from a sulphur process which takes place in the hair, a sulphur process which is particularly strong in people with red hair. And we should note that these things are exceptionally interesting. I did indeed become acquainted with people where one could say that it meant something that they were fiery with their flaming red hair. There was an exceptionally strong real sulphur process, whereas black hair has a relatively strong iron process in it. Now consider that this is the product of the whole human organization. In the one instance we have a human being who constantly produces something that is an intensive combustible material, sulphur, so that it penetrates into his hair. In the other instance he secretes something which is iron, which does not burn at all but is something different. That shows a fundamental difference between the two people with regard to their organization. So something that is roughly the case in general is also the case specifically in each person with regard to their hair so that you can recognize the whole human being from the composition of their hair. How, then, would it be possible not to understand human beings from the structure of their iris? But now you have to consider that these things require the highest level of knowledge, not the ridiculous knowledge which diagnosticians possess about the iris. That, of course, is crude. Particularly in these things that are based on real foundations, the path only leads to true knowledge when we reach the end of it, just as in astrology the path only leads to spirit knowledge at the end whereas before that it is terribly amateurish. The same applies to palmistry and graphology.

Graphology requires real Inspiration. The way people write is a very individual thing; at best we can give some guidance about it. But that guidance will be very rough. Here, too, the same applies as I said before. It does truly require Inspiration in order to draw conclusions about a person from graphology. Now the peculiar thing about graphology is that the handwriting of a person in the present tells us about their state seven years previously. That is an additional factor so that the person who wants to draw conclusions about the present state of a person has to take a detour, has to pass through the whole development again. He arrives at the inner state seven years ago, can then, if he has the vision, follow the path with what he perceived seven years ago and thus has a more thorough knowledge than he would otherwise have.

A similar thing as with the hair and iris applies to what is observed by palmistry. But here, too, you have to have Inspiration, not the superficial rules which are normally given. Palmistry in turn requires a special, a very special facility which maybe one or two people possess in order to investigate the lines of the hands. The latter are indeed intimately connected with human development. All you need to do is compare the lines on your own hands, what the lines of the left and the right hand look like. You see, in general life it is so that people write with their right hand and not with their left. A difference exists. With regard to the lines of the hand this difference is that we can see a person's whole karma in his left hand, if we are so inspired. In the right hand we see the personal capability which that person has obtained in this life. His destiny created this earth life and his capability leads him into the future. There is more to all these things than people think but it is exceptionally dangerous to speak about them in public because we enter territory in which seriousness and charlatanism exist in close proximity. Our reflections here will naturally still lead on to a number of other things.

You see, my dear friends, what I said yesterday at the end of the session means that being a physician involves truly profound moral soul states simply on the basis of the nature of the world's processes. Because I showed you that true knowledge about a medicine means that it will not work on the person who has that knowledge, that specifically the knowledge about a medicine contains something which means that the person with such knowledge excludes himself or herself from being healed by it. Now the mere chemical knowledge does not, of course, exclude anything because it is not knowledge. But true knowledge does exclude in that way.

Consider the following. The human muscular system is grasped by Imagination, cognitively grasped by Imagination, as I showed yesterday. We learn to understand what is at work in the muscles by moving to pictorial imaginative cognition. But if we want to know what has a healing effect in a muscular organ the therapeutic knowledge also has to be imaginative. True knowledge of an internal organ is obtained through Inspiration; that is the only form of true knowledge, chemical knowledge isn't. But let us now assume that you know that a medicine acts on the human muscular system in some way; you have that knowledge by imaginative means. But imaginative knowledge is not like knowledge as we think of it today, because the knowledge we think of today does not penetrate very deeply into a person; it really only exists in the head whereas all imaginative knowledge simultaneously involves the human muscular system. Therapeutic imaginative knowledge is such, my dear friends, that you feel such knowledge in your muscles. You simply have to take these things properly seriously.

In order to make myself perfectly understood, I would like to go as far as to say something paradoxical about the matter. But this paradoxical thing is the truth. My *Philosophy of Freedom*[23] has been little understood because people did not understand how to read it. They read it like any other book, but my *Philosophy of Freedom* is not meant like other books. My *Philosophy of Freedom* begins by living in the thoughts, but in really experienced thoughts. Thoughts which are not experienced, abstract, logical thoughts which are generally prevalent in science today, are experienced in the brain. Such thoughts as I expressed in my *Philosophy of Freedom*—now we get to the paradoxical part—are experienced by the whole human being in the skeletal system, properly as a whole human being in the skeletal system. And I want to say something even more paradoxical—something that has happened of course, only you took no notice of it because you did not connect the two things. If people have understood my *Philosophy of Freedom* they have dreamt several times of skeletons while they were reading it and particularly after they were finished. That is connected morally with the whole position of the *Philosophy of Freedom* with regard to freedom in the world. Freedom already exists when we set the human muscles in motion in the world using the bones. The unfree person follows his drives and instincts. The free person is guided by the demands and requirements of the world which he must first love. He must establish a relationship with this world. That comes to expression in the imagination of the skeletal system. Inwardly it is the skeletal system which experiences the thoughts we experience. So experienced thoughts are experienced in the skeletal system with the whole human being, namely with the whole solidly physical human being. There have been people who wanted to paint pictures from my books; they showed me all kinds of things. They wanted to present the thoughts in the *Philosophy of Freedom* in pictorial form. If we want to paint the content of these thoughts by such means we have to present dramatic scenes that are carried out by human skeletons. Just as freedom itself is something in connection with which we have to jettison everything of a purely instinctive nature, so what people experience when they have thoughts of freedom is something for which they have to jettison their flesh and blood. They have to become skeleton, earthlike, their thoughts truly have to become earthlike. That does mean that we have to work our own way out of it.

I mention this so that you can see that even in ordinary thoughts something happens in which the whole human being is taken hold of. If we move from the thought to Imagination we experience our imagination in the muscular system. We experience Inspiration inwardly in our own organs. Only in the case of Inspiration we should never forget the saying 'naturalia non sunt turpia'.[24] Because it can happen that the most wonderful inspirations are experienced with the kidneys or other lower organs. So higher knowledge really does make demands on the whole human being; and anyone who does not know that imagining is work that is very similar to physical work, because it strains the muscles like real physical work, can have no idea of Imagination and Inspiration. Hence there is also a correlation between physical work and Imagination. If I may mention something personal for example, I have always found that it made a huge contribution to my imagining that I chopped wood as a boy, lifted potatoes, worked with a spade, sowed and did similar things. Well, I do not want to boast about these things but having done them makes it easier to work the muscles hard to facilitate imagining, just like being used to any particular thing makes that thing easier. That is how it is if you have exercised muscles in your youth and if you want to imagine later on. But you see, movements that are not work are of no use. Playing as such is of no benefit for imagining. I do not want to say anything against play, you only need to look at my educational things to see that I have nothing against play, but imagining creates a similar experience in the resting muscle—because it has to be done at rest, of course—as real physical work.

So you can see, as you learn about these admittedly curious things in context here with us on your way to being a physician, how knowledge of these therapeutic things intervenes in your muscular system—and that is something that will be of importance in your karma. Let us assume, for example, that you become familiar with—I am constructing a purely hypothetical case—let us say the real treatment for smallpox. Real smallpox provokes a very strong inspiration, even including Intuition, and what you truly know by this means, my dear friends, if you are real therapists in this field, has a much stronger effect on you if it is true knowledge than vaccination. It has a much stronger effect in a different sense; and in studying the treatment of smallpox as a physician you will cause a kind of preventive healing in yourself and in that way will prepare yourself, if you understand the connection, to be among smallpox sufferers without fear in complete love. But all these things in turn have their reverse side. Because, you see, what you acquire as knowledge of a medicine is, if it is truly imaginative or inspired knowledge, a real medicine; it has healing forces within it. It does not even need to be your own imagination but only one which someone else has, and that is something everyone can do, as I keep repeating. Having the idea of a medicine is effective but it is only effective for as long as you are fearless—because fear is the opposite pole from love. If you go into a sickroom with fear all your therapy will be of no help. If you enter it with love you can disregard yourself, indeed, you can focus with all of your soul on those whom you have to heal, can live in love in your imaginative, inspired knowledge. Then, you see, you will not be involved in the healing process out of a personal quality, as this fearful person with knowledge, but as a loving person with knowledge. Thus medicine is driven towards morality not just from outside but also from inside.

And thus something applies to a high degree in the field of medicine which applies in all fields where we are dealing with spiritual knowledge: we have to develop courage. As you know, courage is what surrounds us everywhere. The air is illusion, courage is what surrounds us everywhere. If we want to live in the world in which we breathe we need to develop courage. If we are cowardly in some way we do not live in the world, we exclude ourselves; we only appear to breathe. The thing you need above all else to study medicine is courage, the courage to heal. It truly is the case that if you have the courage to heal an illness that in itself is the right outlook which in 90 per cent of cases will lead to the correct result, because it is so that these moral qualities are most intimately connected with the process of healing. That is why it should be as follows. First course for medical students: those things which I set out in the first three sessions, creating a basis through obtaining a greater or lesser knowledge of nature and human beings, of the cosmos and human beings. Then the second course: esoteric deepening regarding the action of medical powers, looking at medicine in the way I did in the fourth session and in what I will discuss tomorrow. Then there has to be a final course which must essentially aim to look at treatment in the context of the development of the proper moral abilities by physicians, because the one thing must support the other. And if the final medical course contains what is morally qualified in this way, then disease will truly become the opposite for the physician to what it is for the patient. It becomes something which the physician loves, not in the sense of nurturing it so that the patient remains ill for as long as possible but which he loves because the disease only acquires its meaning when it is healed. What does that mean?

You see, my dear friends, being healthy means bearing the spiritual qualities, the so-called normal soul and spiritual qualities within one. But being ill, having some kind of illness, means actually being influenced by a spiritual quality. I know, of course, that if one of the clever people of our time hears what I am saying now he will say: Aha, here comes the old teaching of possession. Well, it is arguable whether the old teaching of possession is worse than the new one, whether one is possessed by spirits or germs. That is something the value of which still needs to be investigated. Modern physicians always declare themselves in favour of possession in their medical teaching, only it is more appropriate for their understanding to teach about materialistic possession. But it is the case that when we have an illness we have a spiritual quality in us which is not present in the normal course of a person's life. But it is a spiritual quality.

There is another paradox I must mention. Let us assume that you want to understand the connection—I am speaking about a very real fact here—between the elements of the zodiac: Aries, Taurus, Gemini, Cancer, Leo, Virgo, Libra, Scorpio, Sagittarius, Capricorn, Aquarius, Pisces. Now there is a colossal difference between these seven constellations (top) and these five constellations (bottom). If you rise up to Imagination, you get a being that appears to be male for these seven constellations and a being that appears to be female for these five constellations so that in actual fact male-female spreads out over the zodiac in a closed serpentine form in the imaginative perception. Well, no one can receive this imagination without going through the following. Imagine smallpox, which reveals itself in the symptoms of the

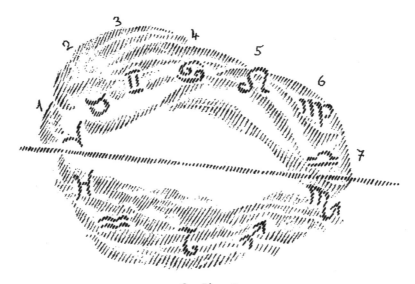

See Plate 8

physical body. But imagine if the following were possible. Imagine a person suffering from smallpox who would have the strength in his astral body and I-organization to draw out the whole of the smallpox disease and only experience it in the astral body and I so that at that moment his physical body was cured. Assume that this were hypothetically possible. What I have set out here cannot happen but if you want to have this imagination you must, without your physical and etheric body taking it on, go through the same thing as I set out hypothetically with regard to smallpox. You have to suffer smallpox in your astral body and I-organization free of the physical and etheric body. In other words, you have to spiritually experience a spiritual correlate of physical illness. Smallpox, my dear friends, is the physical reflection of the state of the I-organization and astral body when you have such an imagination. Now you will understand that in smallpox the influence is simply at work in human beings themselves which with spiritual insight becomes the heavenly imagination.

Here you can see how closely being ill is related to the spiritual life and not to the physical body. Illness is the physical imagination of the spiritual life. And because the physical imagination should not be there, because it should not imitate certain spiritual processes, something can be a disease in the physical organization which in the spiritual world might be of the highest order.

We therefore have to understand illness in such a way that we say: if it were not possible through certain things which we will examine tomorrow to fetch down certain spiritual beings to where they do not belong, they would not be present in the spiritual world either. That shows how closely real spiritual knowledge and illness are related. We actually already recognize the illness when we recognize the spirit. We cannot do anything else. Once we have such a heavenly imagination we know what the disease of smallpox is because it is only the physical projection of our spiritual experience. That basically applies to all our knowledge about illness. We might say that when heaven—or hell, of course—take too strong a hold of a person he becomes ill. If they only take hold of his soul or spirit he becomes wise or clever or insightful.

These are things which you, my dear friends, will have to digest in your soul. Then you will understand the task of anthroposophy as it relates to being a physician because anthroposophy reveals the correct divine archetypes of what is demonically reflected in the diseases. But that can lead you deeper and deeper into the knowledge that the reform of medical studies which is necessary today must be sought on the ground of anthroposophy.

LECTURE 8

My dear friends,

It is, of course, only possible to refer to some things aphoristically here, which in the course of time you will inevitably come across in one way or another if what you have experienced here finds its corresponding continuation in your connection with the medical movement at the Goetheanum.

It should, after all, be emphasized that there can be no healing in opposition to karma. A physician's attitude must essentially be that we cannot heal in opposition to karma. A physician must face in two directions in his attitude with regard to even the most basic question of the intent to heal. The one direction is the unassailable will that karma be fulfilled. A physician needs this will that karma be fulfilled above all with regard to himself because you have seen, my dear friends, that what the physician uses for his patients loses its efficacy in a certain way when applied to himself. It is true that it can in turn be transformed to work for himself. But right now it is enough for you to know what I have said about it. The physician does, of course, also remain subject to karma with regard to his health. But as soon as the attitude exists which I have spoken about, when therapeutic knowledge penetrates the soul as deeply as I said, then we can say that the awareness of karma is increasingly transformed into the pure revelation of karma. Karma has two sides. On the one hand you have to look at karma in such a way that in the sequence of lives on earth you relate your destiny to your previous one. In such a case karma is the expression of the product of your previous lives on earth. But you also have to think of karma directly in the fifth or sixth following life on earth, in the life on earth that follows this one five or six lives away. What is happening now will have consequences then; that is when you will see the final result. If you think this thought properly to the end, it will be clear to you that karma is also something in development, that what is happening now adds something to karma. We can say that our deeds redirect karma in a certain way in one or another direction. Anyone who understands karma cannot be a fatalist.

The one direction is that of karma. It provides firmness and security in life, it provides a firm standpoint. But the other direction is this one, that the will to heal must exist. This will must never be compromised. It must always work therapeutically in such a way that we can say we have done everything possible even if we are of the opinion that the patient cannot be healed. Such an opinion must be suppressed, everything must be done to heal the patient. I simply allude to that aphoristically.

The most important thing today is that we continue to study esoterically those things which cause our soul forces to awaken in our medical studies. And here you have to consider that for the physician the content of such esoteric knowledge must indeed entail a special activity, assume a specific form. It will simply not be enough for the physician to look at things as they are looked at in normal life and as is done today in normal science. Science does not appeal to the special soul forces which human beings do not have in normal life but, on the contrary, places great value on not appealing to such soul forces. But such general perceptions are not enough for any substance or process in the world to reveal its healing powers. Things only reveal their healing powers when we approach them with certain soul forces which have been awoken. It is now up to you to awaken those soul forces step by step so that things talk to you about the way in which they can help human beings through you, through your medical knowledge. But in order for that to happen it is important that what I have told you in the last few days about the attitude of the physician is deepened much, much more in your souls.

Let me make a simple observation in the way that it should really be made in a medical course. Here it will be aphoristic but if there is enough time the matter will not be aphoristic but will develop naturally before the soul of the medical student.

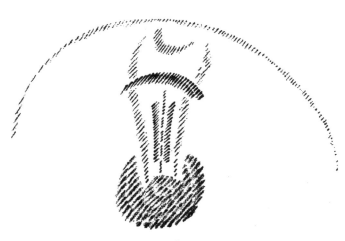

See Plate 9

Take a look at what is revealed through the shape of the bony calvarium. We can draw an outline of it. Look at what is revealed in the shape of the bony calvarium and contrast it with what is revealed to you when you look at a long bone, let us say the femur, which I will draw in outline. Now these things do not exist in isolation but the bony calvarium has the various physical forces surrounding it. Equally the long bone has various forces around it. But when you look at this long bone it will never reveal its essence to you other than if you look at it in the context of the whole of the cosmos. Now imagine that here we have the long bone; its forces pass along its length and point towards the centre of the earth when human beings acquire the physical posture they need to develop. But that is not the most important thing. The most important thing is that it aligns these forces with the axis between the centre of the earth and the moon. So those things which are aligned like the femoral long bone or the upper arm, or like the muscles in those locations, are integrated into the forces that connect the earth with the moon.

You can imagine it like this. Here you have the earth and forces flare up from the earth towards the moon. And everything is harnessed into these forces which has the alignment of, let us say, the femur when the human being stands or walks. In contrast, all those things which are positioned like the calvarium are arranged to coincide with the move-

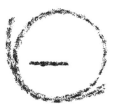

See Plate 9

ment of Saturn. The rotational forces of Saturn are at work in them, so that we can say: human beings are formed from below upwards through the connection between earth and moon; they are closed off through what lies in the rotational force of Saturn. But both types of force are in opposition. If you look at the former forces, those which lie in the connection between the earth and the moon, then these forces contain everything which gives human beings their sculpted form, which builds them up three-dimensionally. We might say that these forces contain a secret sculptor who builds up the human being three-dimensionally whereas there is constant catabolism in the other forces. In the latter the matter which builds up human beings sculpturally is dispersed again. So when you cut your nails you are in the Saturn forces with your scissors. When you eat, then the direction of this component—it is characterized by the direction away from the earth—is towards the moon. All forces aligned with the direction of the moon are anabolic. All forces aligned with the direction of Saturn disperse the human being; and the human soul, the human spirit lies in this interchange between being dispersed and being sculpturally built up. That is how they reveal themselves.

Now the things which are external and the things which human beings have within themselves, connected with the etheric body, they are linked to these peripheral forces. Silver reveals itself to be connected with the anabolic forces in certain respects so that when you notice that the anabolic forces in human beings are being overwhelmed by the catabolic forces you can correct this development, as a rule, with a medicine which is based on silver. But if you notice that the anabolic forces are running wild, that they are holding the human form together and are preventing it from scattering, as we might say, then you will always see that we have to make use of medicines which are connected with Saturn, which are connected with lead. So if we can understand how a human being is structured, we can have an understanding of how we have to act.

It is a matter of getting into such a way of observation. Now you see, my dear friends, the true world, the world of the spirit, lies somewhere of which it has rightly always been said that it is beyond a threshold; human beings are on this side of the threshold. It is indeed necessary that human beings should cross this threshold to come to a true understanding, a true insight into the constitution of the cosmos. It is, however, generally dangerous for human beings to cross this threshold without any preparation. Because if human beings suffuse normal sensory perception with the kind of thoughts they have in ordinary life and take these with them into the spiritual world across the threshold, they produce real phantasmagoria by judging things beyond the threshold in the same way as they do here. And that is why there is the spiritual being at the threshold from whom we can learn that we require completely different concepts when we cross the threshold, that phantasmagoria will make us incapable of action if we enter the spiritual world with our ordinary concepts taken from the sensory world. This Guardian of the Threshold is truly there to warn us that we must first obtain the ideas that we need in the spiritual world. People do not normally believe that the concepts that are of use in the spiritual world are unusually different from the concepts that are of use here in the physical world. In the physical world, for example, a part is always smaller than the whole. That is deemed to be an axiom. It is not like that in the spiritual world. There the part is always larger than the whole. You can learn that using the example of the human being. If we assume a force which human beings possess, for example, when they build up their body from the mineral component, and if we look at the forces at work in any part of the human being, then those things which form the organs, in other words, that part of the human being, is significantly greater from a cosmic perspective than the human being as a whole. It is not so easy for you to picture the idea that the part is greater than the whole because you are used to the sensory world, but that is indeed the case with regard to the supersensory world. Hence we have to reach a point where we recognize the possibility that in the spiritual world the part can be greater than the whole. None of our mechanics and physics applies in the spiritual world but the direct opposite. Here in the sensory world a straight line is the shortest path between two points. In the spiritual world it is the longest because if you proceed in a straight line you have to overcome the greatest number of obstacles. Every other direction is shorter than a straight line. We have to be quite clear that if we want to enter the spiritual world we need the opposite concepts to what is commonplace in the physical world in order to avoid confusion when we enter the spiritual world. That requires courage. We have to have the courage to cross the spiritual threshold, to cross that gulf. If we go through that whole thing, crossing over into the spiritual world, passing the Guardian of the Threshold and arriving on the other side, if we go through that in our soul and spirit, consciously in our astral body and I, then everything is well. But if we do not go through that cleanly in our I and astral body then an illusion is created and when this illusion in turn affects the human being, illness arises. So whenever there is some kind of illness in a person, he or she really has the Guardian of the Threshold within himself or herself—but in a kind of demonic reflection.

So I return to the demonic about which I have already had to speak. And why is that? That is because if we look at the human being with ordinary perceptions, everything becomes mixed up. On the one side we have the I and astral body and on the other side the etheric body and physical body. And all of them are mixed up when we look at them ordinarily. So it is very important that we learn to differentiate the soul element in human beings from the physical. When the soul is in the body and you look at the human being, the soul does not appear as what it really is. The soul in reality is indeed light. And you will increasingly have to understand that the human soul, when looked at separately from the body, is light. Among those elements, those etheric elements with which it is associated, it belongs to light. The human soul absolutely belongs to the realm of light. We see it correctly if we see it as part of light.

By contrast, the body is associated with weight. Now I explained how weight is overcome, how the brain becomes a lot lighter than it would be outside. But the way that the body is organized, as we perceive it in its essence, it is associated with weight. Just as you get hydrogen and oxygen if you analyse water chemically, you have to divide the human being into the soul with its luminous power and the body with the impact of its weight.

These two entities, the soul with its luminous power and the body with the impact of its weight, are confusingly intermingled when we look at them with ordinary eyes. Because of that we cannot identify the nature of the illness from looking at the body. If you organize your soul so that it can look at the human being in such a way that the nature of the illness can be revealed, and if you understand by that means how the nature of the illness can be recognized, then the nature of the healing forces in lead and in silver will be revealed to you. But you have to take this medical life incredibly seriously and develop your meditative life with such strength in your soul that you learn to see the world, to take hold of the world differently. And that is why I now want to give you something to take away with you which, properly meditated, my dear friends, and added to the other things, will lead you to obtain the kind of relationship with special substances which these substances them-selves have to the healthy and sick human being. You have to look at what I am about to write on the blackboard[*] as awakening the per-ception in your soul that what you see of the human being in normal life is not the reality, but that the reality is what you see when you bring to life in your soul what lies in these words. Then you will see the truth of the human being in the relationship between the one and the other.

So far I have spoken in such a way that you can understand the human being in general in his or her relationship with the cosmos. Today I want to inscribe into your soul something that will enable you to take a tiny piece of gold and look at it meditatively. I beat it into a thin leaf and thus get something greenish when I look through it like this. It looks greenish. Its greenish appearance awakens the same inner experience that is aroused by a green meadow, the green plant cover of the earth—not just in some vague analogy but in a precise way because I approach the gold leaf with deeper powers of the soul. But by immersing myself properly with my soul powers in the small translucent gold leaf, the opposing soul power is also awoken. And because I have the greenish shimmering gold leaf here I do not just get a contrasting

---

[*] This blackboard has not been preserved.

effect—as physiological physicists would say—but this contrasting effect contains a whole world, the impression of a shimmering world just as everything shimmers around me in a reddish matt and bluish red light. At that moment I know that the whole world lies in this small piece of gold. And this small piece of gold which I hold in my hand, which shimmers in a greenish colour here, is actually a whole sphere. It has been compressed into this small atomistic leaf. I cannot have a piece of gold without it being a whole sphere, without it being a node for a whole sphere so that I learn to live in the bluish red and the bluish purple of a sphere. And when you become familiar with other characteristics of gold, then you will learn to connect these other characteristics in a living way with what you receive in a kind of soul vision. You will, for example, experience in a thorough, a fundamental way the characteristic with which you are familiar, that gold does not tolerate being combined with oxygen. You will say to yourselves: human beings live because they have oxygen, because they constantly process oxygen. In the etheric body—you saw it for yourselves—everything is different. The latter is connected with what is not anchored in the physical body. Gold is connected with the etheric body because it does not tolerate being combined with oxygen, so that precisely through this one characteristic gold has a healing effect in the etheric body with regard to all those things which oxygen can cause in the physical body. Thus gold is a medicine that can act properly from the centre of the human being. The inner truth of the words 'gold is sun' is revealed to you in the shining impression of the matt blue, reddish light. It is wholly sun. So here you have this one node which simply indicates that in the cosmos gold is sun and that gold-sun is related to the etheric body.

You see, such observations lead you to understand the characteristics of substances which are required for therapy. But you will only achieve this if you take seriously not as external words but as a constant inner challenge to the soul:

See in your soul
    Luminous power
Feel in your body the
    Might of gravity

That has to be truly practised. You must practise it as if your soul were to become something which truly expands outwards, which is flowing light, luminous power; and your body could become something which through its own inner longing for gravity combines itself with the interior of the earth. You truly have to experience this incredible contrast, then you will separate soul and body which have to be separated. Then it continues:

> Spirit Self shines out
> > In luminous power

That is the only way you will understand the whole. Because the human I blossoms in the soul as an inner experience. Hence you also have to understand the image of the I arising in the soul striving outwards luminously into the cosmos.

> The strength of God's spirit is
> > Contained in the might of gravity

It truly was not just a superficial image, my dear friends, but something that corresponded to a deep truth when people in earlier times referred to the human body as a temple for the divine. And as much as it is true that the I rules in the soul when the soul is conscious, it is equally true that the Deity rules in the body. You must not address your body as your own because the body does not belong to the human being, the body belongs to God. That is how it is. The human body grows out of divine forces, only the soul within it belongs to the human being so that you have truly to see your body as the temple of God.

And it is incredibly important to know:

> Spirit Self shines out
> > In luminous power

—of the soul—

> The strength of God's spirit is
> > Contained in the might of gravity

God's spirit is contained in the human body just like the I in the human soul.

But now we get to the important thing:

> But luminous power
>> Must not
> Take hold of the
>> Might of gravity

When human beings are asleep, it will be obvious to you that they have the soul entity and the physical body in separation. They are then separate in human beings. In that situation the soul does not take hold of the body. But when human beings are awake it also holds good that, although the astral body and I are immersed in the physical and etheric body, there is still an inner division, an inner separation of luminous power and the might of gravity. What must not happen is that a component develops chemically consisting of luminous power and the might of gravity; they have to be inwardly separate. They must not mix mechanically or, indeed, combine inwardly. They have to act in parallel in the same space—the might of the body's weight downwards, the luminous power of the soul upwards. That is why the following words are important:

> But luminous power
>> Must not
> Take hold of the
>> Might of gravity
> And neither must the
>> Might of gravity
> Penetrate
>> Luminous power

Those are the opposites. So in reality, my dear friends, those things which our sensory knowledge continuously mixes up must exist as separate entities in the human being. If you look at the human being externally with sensory knowledge everything is mixed up. And if human beings were what normal perception sees them to be, they would always be ill. Human beings can be healthy but our perception, our sensory perception, of human beings is always of illness. We always see human beings as ill but that is, of course, always maya, illusion.

Because in their true self human beings must never be as we see them. In their true being luminous power and the might of gravity must never be mixed up. They must be inwardly separate from one another. So it must not be as happens in the case of water where hydrogen and oxygen form a chemical compound and really disappear as such. In human beings that only happens through sensory perception; the latter has produced the absurdity of having taken on a chemical view and looking at human beings as if they were a compound of luminous power and the might of gravity. They are separate and must remain separate—as if hydrogen and oxygen were always separate in water despite being in it together.

> Because if luminous power
> Takes hold of the might of gravity

—that is, if luminous power really enters the might of gravity—

> Because if luminous power
> Takes hold of the might of gravity
> And if the might of gravity penetrates
> Luminous power
> Then in cosmic error
> Soul and body combine
> To destruction

—the destruction is illness.

As I said, you have to take these things in all seriousness to such an extent that it forms your body, that you can truly look at the human being and see luminous power and the might of gravity and that you have the feeling that they are hostile to one another when they come into contact. They come into contact in illness. And when luminous power takes a hold of the might of gravity, the physical illnesses arise; when the might of gravity penetrates luminous power, the so-called psychiatric illnesses arise. Because remember what there is. Remember that the spirit of God lives in the body. So when luminous power takes hold of the might of gravity the human being is illegitimately appropriating God.

Now, to think about and penetrate with your feelings all these things with the necessary moral impulse and then to want them with what you have felt—that will teach you gradually to look at the things and processes in the world in a real way. It will give you an idea how to separate luminous power from the might of gravity when the latter has been gripped by the former by using something that will support the etheric body from the astral body through an external substance or a process in the human being. You see, if you penetrate something like that properly with the feelings in your soul, then you will also gain insight into what it is that heals in eurythmy therapy. Because the healing aspect in eurythmy therapy is fundamentally that element which takes particular account of cosmic forces in its healing action. When you do eurythmy therapy exercises with consonants, you are in the moon forces. When you develop eurythmy therapy forces using vowels, you are in the Saturn forces. So when doing eurythmy therapy human beings directly feel their way into the cosmos with these two types of forces. It is like this, for example. Let us assume we could determine—because the key thing in medicine is of course the therapy, but there is no therapy if we do not have a usable diagnosis—let us assume we could determine that the structural element is too strong in a person, that he has salt and carbohydrate structures within him which he cannot overcome: there is too much structure. If you take a real look at the more subtle effects on the organism—the symptoms can occur unobtrusively—eurythmy using vowels which counter such structures can have an exceptionally beneficial effect. Or let us assume that a small child begins to show a tendency to stammer. Well, I certainly do not want to draw any unprofessional conclusions about some cause or other of the stammer; there can, of course, be a whole range of disorders. But in all situations the disorders associated with a stammer work in such a way that there is a predominating structural force and that is why vowel exercises are used in eurythmy therapy for a stammer. And they can be used in the sequence, the form in which the vowels naturally come to expression in the human being. So we can indeed achieve an exceptional amount in children who show signs of a stammer with eurythmy therapy simply with the normal vowel sequence a, e, i, o, u if we have the necessary perseverance and love.

If you reflect on all these things, my dear friends, then you will realize that it is important for you to think of the esoteric background that I gave you a few days ago and just now as a kind of moral underpinning of your medical studies. By moral I mean a feeling of commitment to an obligation, a feeling of commitment to establish the required constant mood in the soul through meditation so that you encounter the world in the right way. If we had a year for these lectures we would be able to go into much greater detail, which would then stand you in good stead in practice. But as we have only been able to give an introduction to all these things, my dear friends, it is particularly important to begin by speaking about the development of the medical powers in the human being, to give you these medical hints in particular. Because if you now embark on your medical studies with these esoteric hints you will see things will be different. However, they might be even more difficult. When a person of today with a somewhat dull mind—people's minds today are already dulled in primary school, something which is reinforced in secondary school, and then they go on to university— when such a person with a dull mind starts to study medicine he might survive the first or second year through a certain inner stubbornness if through his social background he feels some moral whip driving him on. But he will not become a physician. He will become a person employed by society to pretend to be a physician, but he will not be a physician. Now you will, of course, develop a subtle power of soul through letting such things act on your soul powers. And sometimes the way that psychology and physiology and pathology—which form the basis of medicine—act on you will be painful. It will truly feel as if sometimes you are given stones instead of bread. But you will nevertheless be able to obtain something even from those stones by yourselves. And the things provided will still to a certain degree be relevant. You will be able to learn something despite the difficult path on which you have embarked. There is no alternative because at present the world with its materialism is still very powerful and we have to work in it in one way or another. We have to work out of the situation in which we find our- selves when we are part of the world.

And so you have to become physicians in the way that the world demands and suffuse your medical studies with what you can obtain from here. And that is why I want to repeat once more: you will indeed, my dear friends, have the opportunity to come together, to connect in the way that I have spoken about. You should have complete confidence in the way that the Medical Section at the Goetheanum is managed by me together with Dr Wegman. It is precisely the kind of medicine which can be researched here which can show you—forgive the paradoxical way of putting it—how it can truly be experienced in human life here. You will be able to receive it and so what you must do once you are out in the world again, when something or other occurs to you, is to write to us with your wishes, your heart's desires. And what the one person writes will receive an answer which will be sent to everyone in the monthly newsletter. In this way your external medical studies will be suffused by the means available at this time with those things which we can provide today.

You see, basically there are still exceptionally few people—they can really only be young people—who can build a bridge between the spiritual intentions of Dornach and what holds materialistic power out in the world. It can only be a few people at the moment and really only those who are engaged in their studies. Why? What you initially hear as coming from Dornach in various fields would be nonsense if it actually were from Dornach. On one occasion when I had to give a lecture to a group of students about a particular chapter of therapy all the students from the whole faculty were there as well as a full professor, a real professor. Now you see, my dear friends, I could see that he came to the lecture because he wanted to find confirmation for his belief that I would talk a lot of rubbish, as medical amateurs do. It was a study in metamorphosis to see how on the one hand he became increasingly annoyed inwardly but on the other hand experienced astonishment. Because he had to concede that it was not rubbish, but he could not, of course, acknowledge that because that would completely contradict what he had for decades considered to be true and accurate. Indeed, the most one could expect from that gentleman was—I spoke to him afterwards when it became clear—that he would refuse to come anywhere near the subject. He would not have needed to steer well clear of it if he had seen that it was rubbish. Then he could easily have made the usual disparaging remarks. He also thought that he could easily do it, but he couldn't, and so the most one could ask of a professor like that was that he would refuse to come near the subject. You could not demand more of him. But young people have to adopt quite a different attitude. They do not yet carry all that baggage with them. So they can come to grips with these things for the benefit of humankind. And when that begins to happen, my dear friends, then we will reach a point at which gradually—perhaps faster than we think—the Goetheanum's spirituality will become part of medicine.

But as matters stand, we have to begin by continuing in all seriousness with the way in which—as Dr Wegman said—you approached her so that we can establish in full trust the connection with those things of which in reality a true medical course should consist, a medical course which has to flow into today's general materialistic medicine. You can do a lot for yourselves in this respect, but also a lot for the world and sick humanity, if you consider the things you have heard now not as something ephemeral but as the starting point for those things in which you have made such an exceptionally positive beginning. In this spirit, my dear friends, let us remain united, let us remain united in such a way that you retain your centre in Dornach here at the Goetheanum and truly adhere to that centre so that it can be active through you in the world. That is what I wish to give you to take away with you like a kind of reminder, I might say. Then things will turn out well, then other things will follow from what we have discussed and experienced here. You can have a feeling what that ideal should be in a beautiful way, but you can also turn it into a real way of life.

So, my dear friends, that is what we will do.[25]

> See in your soul
>> Luminous power
> Feel in your body the
>> Might of gravity
> Spirit Self shines out
>> In luminous power
> The strength of God's spirit is
>> Contained in the might of gravity
> But luminous power
>> Must not

Take hold of the
    Might of gravity
And neither must the
    Might of gravity
Penetrate
    Luminous power
Because if luminous power
    Takes hold of the might of gravity
And if the might of gravity penetrates
    Luminous power
Then in cosmic error
    Soul and body combine
To destruction

EASTER COURSE

LECTURE 9

DORNACH, 21 APRIL 1924

M_Y dear friends,
At the meeting which we held here after the Christmas course we let
those things act on us which can deepen medicine esoterically. And in
the way in which this can be done, of course, in such a short meeting we
attempted to find the greatest possible access to the esoteric aspect of
medicine as appears appropriate particularly for those younger people
who are making their way in medicine. We also assimilated within
ourselves in individual formulas those things which can produce a
medical attitude in order to work on them further, and we emphasized
how necessary such a medical attitude is. Now I assume, my dear
friends, that you have worked inwardly on these things for some time. I
do not, of course, imagine such work to consist of sitting there and
considering them theoretically but that now and again, when we feel the
inner need, we let these things work on our soul and allow the soul to
develop. Now the way in which we dealt with these things at the time
meant that a particular fact occurred which, I believe, is of importance
for the future. The intensely compressed way in which the esoteric
matter was presented at the time in a certain sense inevitably created in
one or the other person a more or less great need to look at certain inner
difficulties. The things which are given esoterically do not always exist
to make life as easy as possible for us but in a certain way the opposite
applies. They are indeed also there to make life difficult for us, to take us
into the difficulties of understanding the world, the way we perceive the
world and the human being, so that when we become aware of those

difficulties we take the opposite path of development to the one which is so often pursued in our culture—namely the opposite to the superficial path of development. We can immerse ourselves in the soul only if we become aware of the difficulties which exist between the external world and human beings. And so I think the best thing to do on this occasion is for you to reflect on those inner difficulties, raise them in the form of questions and we can then focus our discussion on those things which will further advance our cause. To begin with, I would ask you to tell me from within your group what inner or outer difficulties have arisen. Practitioners will have experienced difficulties, students will have experienced difficulties. There are a number of people among us who are nearing the end of their studies—they will have experienced very special difficulties. We will resolve that by seeking for a solution. Everyone has also received the first newsletter[26] and will have seen that there is still a great deal to be said in response to specific questions. I would like to ask whether someone has a question. It can be as specific or general as you like—it will undoubtedly lead us on to other things. But such questions will allow us to get away from the lecture-style into something we can experience.

Ernst Harmstorf:[27] Asks about the course of the year; Calendar of the Soul and certain constellations of the stars.

That is not necessary. You mean the observations of the constellations of the stars? Yes. Well, it does help if we have the observable constellation of the stars in our consciousness. But if I have understood you correctly you are asking what should happen when we allow what we have received as formulas to work on the soul. It works through its own mantric power, and orienting oneself by the external stars can indeed provide support. But you have to consider the following. Take, for instance, the most obvious example of a human-cosmic connection which can still be observed today. That is the menstrual cycle. It takes its course in such a way that it evidently has cosmic origins, but not in our time—its cosmic origins lie in a much earlier cosmic development in which our earth also participated. Then it became self-contained, emancipated from the cosmos in the course of time so that now there is no longer a direct dependence. We cannot therefore say: moon phases

= menstruation. We cannot say that. But we can very well say: there was once a point at which the one was identical with the other, then they split apart. The moon phases are one thing, menstruation is another. That is the one division. The other one is not guided by the greater moon phases but by the daily ones. Ebb and flood were identical with what happens through the moon. Once again they have separated. The moon goes its way and ebb and flood go their way.

These things also determine the effect of the mantric element. It was indeed once the case that what happened through this in the human being was identical with what happened in the cosmos; the split has now occurred in such a way that we must first have the right orientation. If we want to have such support from outside we have to tell ourselves that what we want to happen inwardly is written in the cosmos. But in reflecting on this we must, however, make ourselves inwardly independent and be able to experience the course of events inwardly for ourselves in emancipation from the course taken by the cosmos. That is why it is not absolutely necessary that the constellations of the stars have to be taken into account in the effect of a mantra just as it is completely out of the question that menstruation is regulated by the external position of the moon because it has become part of our nature. It is equally the case today that all of our inner progression brought about by the mantras must take its course in emancipation from the external cosmos. That, as I have often had to explain in the past in other areas, is the difference between eastern and western esotericism. The eastern person wholly takes the view that human beings have come out of the cosmos and have to return there, have to connect with it again.

Take the posture of the Buddha.[28] It is a return to earlier conditions. His whole posture speaks of that, the crossed legs, the exclusion of the limbs. The position of the arms is also such that the whole relationship with the earth is immobilized. All the things which emancipate us from the cosmos are paralysed. We can see how human beings reintegrate themselves back into the cosmos. They return again. And that is really what all of eastern esotericism is like. It is a move backwards. And our western esotericism can only be a move forwards, an ever greater emancipation. That is why it is not so inwardly easy—particularly when used in specific fields. Of course, if you come across, let us say, a particular pathology and you look at the constellation of the stars and see that the case occurred specifically when, let us say, Saturn stood in opposition to the moon, that does of course have a particular meaning. Because if you then adopt a Saturn and moon approach in your treatment—that means lead and silver in earthly terms (as you know, Saturn = lead, moon = silver), and you tell yourself I will use lead cosmically in the way it has become cosmic in the earth and I will make silver earthly by trying to pulverize, dissolve it, i.e. change it into an earthly state, and thereby call forth the same constellation as is expressed in the heavens through the opposition to the moon—then you can heal in the spirit of the cosmic forces. But at the same time you are putting the person in a situation which throws him or her back to earlier human developmental stages whereas if you simply start directly from what is earthly—the connection of a person with lead and silver—you are already located in something that emancipates itself in the human being and you are not looking at the past but at the future. In that case you will indeed do something similar; but you will achieve it from inside by becoming acquainted with the nature of lead and silver, by knowing that lead works as substance while silver works through what it actually becomes when it is shattered, dissolved, i.e. dissolved into atoms. But you will compare it with already emancipated human nature, not with the cosmos. In this way you do have to find the right mindset; that is why it can be a help to recall the actual constellation of stars. But to begin with you will have to use all your strength to allow your own inner soul impulses to work on you arising from what we have had as mantric formulas, and rather to seek everything from out of your inner self.

Ilse Knauer:[29] What do I have to do from out of the I when I meditate?

You mean from out of the I? Well, as you know, meditation consists of the following. As a modern person, you feel that you have to understand each sentence. That represents the pronounced activity of the I in the present incarnation. Everything you do intellectually is a pronounced activation of the I. The intellect is [predominant] in the present incarnation and everything else is covered up by the I, works upwards in a dreamlike way at best and is unconscious. In contrast, meditating means switching such intellectual endeavour off and, to begin with, taking the content of the meditation as it is given, purely in its wording, if I can put it like that. So if you approach the content of the meditation intellectually, before internalizing it, you activate your I because you have thoughts about the content of the meditation; it is outside you. If you allow the content of the meditation to be present in your consciousness just as it is given, do not reflect on it at all but allow it to be present in your consciousness, then it is not your I from the present incarnation which is at work in you but the one from the previous incarnation. You silence your intellect; you simply immerse yourself in the word content which you hear inwardly, not outwardly, as word content. You immerse yourself in that and in doing so your inner human being, which is not the one of the present incarnation, works in the content of the meditation. But that makes the content of the meditation not something which you should understand but which has a real effect in you, has such a real effect that finally you perceive 'now I have experienced something which I could not experience previously'.

Take a simple meditation content which I have frequently given: 'Wisdom lives in the light'. Well, if you start reflecting on it you can find out a great deal of clever stuff and just as much nonsense about it. It exists to be inwardly heard: 'Wisdom lives in the light'. When you listen to it inwardly in this way, something which is not from the present incarnation but which you have brought with you from the previous one is attentive in you. And it thinks and feels, and after a time something is illuminated in you which you did not know before and which you could not have thought about with your own intellect. You are inwardly much further ahead than your intellect. It only contains a small section of what there is.

You do have to take the things which are generally given in anthroposophy in quite a concrete way, in quite a tangible way. Consider the following. Human beings really renew their whole physical body when the change of teeth occurs. That must be taken as a fundamental fact. Human beings developing a second set of teeth is only the most external symptom, only a part of what is happening. Just as the so-called milk teeth are replaced, the whole of the human organism is replaced so that human beings after the change of teeth have become something completely new in terms of their physical substance when compared to what they were when they were born. The modern view, which muddles everything up, thinks that human beings are born, then they undergo the change of teeth through a metamorphosis, and then they continue to develop.

That is not how it is. This is what happens. Human beings when they are physically born have a body, including the so-called milk teeth, which is the result of heredity. They have received a body which is the result of those things which lie in the whole series of antecedents. That is where the body of the first seven years, if we want to express it in figures, comes from. From the age of seven to 14 they also have a body but that has not come from a transformation of the first one; something intervened here which human beings brought with them to earth. Now you have to think of the matter like this. Human beings have their body. This body, which they have as a result of the hereditary line, is a model—they have it as a model. Now they take earthly substance into this body. Human beings would process this earthly substance which they take into their body in the first seven years in a quite different form if they only worked with the forces which they bring with them from their pre-earthly existence. They would produce something of quite a different nature. When human beings are born, they do not arrive with a tendency to develop a person with eyes, ears, a nose, as they are when they stand here on earth. They arrive with a tendency to form the human being in such a way that they are basically developed very little through their pre-earthly being from out of the head. The greatest care is taken specifically with regard to the rest. Those things which atrophy in embryonic life are developed in the astral sphere, in the I-organization so that we have to say with regard to the physical embryo: the physical part of the embryo has been wonderfully developed but the pre-earthly human being had very little to do with it to begin with.

In contrast, the human being, the pre-earthly human being, is involved to the greatest extent in everything surrounding. The pre-earthly human being lives in that, in what is broken down in the physical sphere and goes away as chorion, amnion and so on. The pre-earthly human being lives in that. [See Plate 10] Now if you imagine it schematically, you can imagine it like this, that the cosmic is recreated to begin with. That is really what human beings want to do when they descend from pre-earthly to earthly existence. Why do they not do it? Because there is a given model. And in accordance with this model they transform what is pre-earthly, using the incorporated substances, during the first seven years. They would actually prefer to create something more spherical and produce a spherically organized human being. But that is transformed in accordance with the model. And so the pre-earthly gives form to this second physical human being, who then exists from the age of seven to 14, out of the pre-earthly forces; but it does so initially by adhering to the model which comes from the hereditary forces.

Now, you see, here you have two force entities in the human being which can really be distinguished. How can we understand these force entities? Take the outline of *Occult Science*[30] to hand, on this occasion from the perspective and with the sentiments of a physician, and read the section in it where the book speaks about the development of the Earth, how we first have Saturn development, [See Plate 10] then Sun development, then we have Moon development, Earth development and so on. If you follow the description of this development there, you will have to say to yourself: up until the Sun everything was one. Not until that point did the Earth and the Sun, the Earth and the Moon separate, so that human beings lived in the cosmos until the middle of this development. They lived in the Sun and Moon as well as in the Earth. Then they lived outside the Sun after the separation of the Sun, outside the Moon after the separation from the Moon. So cosmic forces worked on human nature until the separation of the Sun, also those which today are outside the earth, in the moon, in the sun. They worked in human beings because human beings were part of this world which still included Sun and Moon. After this human beings were subject to development which lay outside Sun and Moon. [See Plate 10 bottom right]

But now the following is the case. Assume a development which contains everything within itself which is earthly today and also those things which belong to the sun and moon; subsequently everything that is from outside the earth emancipated itself from all that is earthly. The earthly part continued along its own path; it dried up, hardened, became physical, and that is what you find today in the hereditary stream, that has become coarse in the hereditary stream. You will find those things which they [human beings] have adopted after the separation of sun and moon in what they owe to the action of the forces from the cosmos—that is the point. So that you obtain a model for creating your second human being, a model which actually represents something ancient and artistic, which your father and mother were able to give you, which could be created when the sun and moon were still combined with the earth. Forces developed at the time which actually give human beings their earthly configuration, because you will easily understand that this human configuration is an earthly one. Imagine for a minute that your self in your essential nature is removed from the earth. What are you to do with it? You would be very unhappy if you had to use something like your legs after death. Legs are only useful if they are subject to the earth's forces of gravity, if we make the legs part of the forces of gravity of the earth. Legs only have a meaning on earth, just like the arms and hands. So a whole part of our organization only makes sense in its present form if we are earth beings. What we are as human beings on earth is useless with regard to the cosmos. That is why we want to form a completely different organization when we arrive on earth as soul and spiritual beings. We want to create an environment, we want to produce all kinds of configurations within this environment, but we do not want this human being which is of no use to us in the cosmos. The latter is only given us as a model and we furnish the second human being in accordance with this model.

That is why in this first period of life we are involved in a constant struggle between what comes from our previous life and what comes from the hereditary development. Those two things are in conflict. And that conflict comes to expression in the childhood diseases. And just think how intimately the whole inner human soul and spiritual existence is connected during early childhood with the physical organization. Just as you can see how the second teeth emerge, how the second tooth ejects the first one, how they are occupied with one another, so the whole second human being is occupied with the first. Except that the supersensory human being is contained in the second human being while an alien earthly model is contained in the former. They work into one another. And if you observe in the right way how they work into one another, then just look at how the inner human being, which was there as soul and spirit in pre-earthly existence, if it has too much of an upper hand for a time has to work into the physical in a particularly strong way, has to adhere to the model with particular intensity and how as a result it causes injury because it collides with it constantly and says: I want get rid of this form—then this struggle is expressed as scarlet fever. If the inner human being is so delicate that it constantly gives way, that it wants to form the substances which are assimilated more in its own image, and if it fights against the model, then this struggle is expressed as measles. And so this mutual struggle comes to expression in the childhood diseases. And we will also only understand what happens later in the right way if we can take these things correspondingly into account.

Of course it is terribly easy for a materialist to say that this is all twaddle because we can see that children look like their parents and grandparents not just up to the change of teeth but also beyond. That is nonsense. Some people just happen to be weaker, are guided more strongly by the hereditary forces, make their second human being more similar to the model, and that is of course what it will look like. But they did that themselves by taking their cue to a greater extent from the model. But we also have people who after the change of teeth become very dissimilar to what they were before. Then the part which comes from the spiritual and soul life before birth is strong and they adhere less to the model. And so it is simply a case of observing these things in the right context. We can see it because everything which has to be absorbed has initially to be absorbed, processed inwardly by the child in such a way that the I and the astral body come into intimate contact with the food. That need no longer be the case later.

Human beings never again get into a situation of having to develop something themselves to such an extent to accord with a model than in the first seven years. In that period they have to process everything they absorb such in their I and astral body that it can recreate the model. So that has to be accommodated and the world has organized things in such a way that milk can come very close to etheric development. Its substantiality is such that it actually still has an etheric body and because the substance, when it is absorbed by the child, still has an organizing action reaching as far as the etheric body, the astral body can intercept the milk so that the intimate contact can arise between that which is absorbed and the astral and I-organization. Hence there is a very profound, intimate relationship between the external food and the inner soul and spiritual organization of the child.

And, you see, now you have to get to the stage as physicians of processing all the things, these strange things, I have told you just now. We can see in the whole way that the child drinks milk how the astral body and I intercept the milk. That can really be seen. Meditate on the mantras, on the one hand, by letting the mantra work on you, so that you release your soul forces. On the other hand, simply meditate on the child. Visualize how the descending soul and spiritual part initially approaches the physical food with the exclusion of the model, and that what then happens between the soul and spiritual part and the food is determined by the forms of the model. If you imagine that properly—the excessive action of the soul and spiritual part—it will be come together for you in the development of scarlet fever. The insufficient action of the soul and spiritual part, which trembles in the face of the model, will be encapsulated for you in the development of measles. If you imagine that meditatively you will turn ordinary meditation into medical meditation. The fact that people want to understand everything today with their reason is a most dreadful thing. You cannot understand anything in medicine with reason. The most you might be able to understand with reason is the diseases of the minerals and we do not cure those. Everything medical in nature has to be grasped with direct perception, which first has to be trained.

You will not be able to observe these things in an adult person. The digestive tract absorbs the foods—that is an inwardly mediated process—whereas in the child the astral body and the I absorb the food; in the latter case there are still unfinished human forms to be organized and developed in accordance with the model. If you meditate on the child you will see a mighty metamorphosis taking place.

You will see how the soul and spiritual element lights up and how food introduces darkness and shadow, how the second human being is

formed in colour, as it were, out of light and darkness. [See Plate 10]
You will be able to see how indeed the pre-earthly part of the human
being is in brightness while the darkness is that part which is ingested as
outer food. A brightness spreads over the darkness in the child which
comes from what is pre-earthly, the milk enters as darkness: they form
the various colours together. What is white on a physical level is black in
the spiritual. The opposite is always the case. That gives you the
opportunity to use your I in quite a different way from the way you
normally use it in life. Just look at the wimpish act which is entailed in
normal intellectual thinking! That is the greatest weakness of human
beings—working intellectually. They only line up one concept after the
other. But if you observe the child in the way I have described here, you
will meditate in such a way that your I-organization is fully involved.
That is something which should also henceforth be taken into account
in our education. In a school like the Waldorf school we have the
children aged from seven to 14: things change in that period, human
beings have developed their second human being. I might see a child
who has been given his or her shape from out of pre-earthly existence in
accordance with the model, which has been thrown off, and now it is of
course the hereditary forces which have been left in the child. They have
been inserted into the model, into the imitation of the model. Now the
child is much too unearthly. For in this case the extraterrestrial part has
been working particularly strongly on the child; now we actually have
the swing of the pendulum in the opposite direction. Previously that
could also be seen externally on human beings, they were completely a
product of their heredity; but now what is externally visible has really
arisen wholly from the inside. Now the external world has to be
acquired. Now that part which only worked with regard to a person's
own human model, totally disregarding the earthly world, has to take
its cue from the external world. Now we have to consider that the astral
body and I-organization between the age of seven and 14 have to work
in such a way that this unearthly being is adapted again to the external
earthly situation. That is concluded with puberty. At that point human
beings have been completely placed within earthly circumstances, have
established their relationship with earthly circumstances and the
earthlike has been integrated into the human being. And so the main

thing in the development of the second human being between the ages of seven and 14 is what he or she brings with him or her from pre-earthly existence which the earthly works into. That reaches its conclusion at puberty and now the third human being is developing. That is why our own karma only begins to work after puberty.

The second human being is substantially shed and the third human being is developed. The latter does not extend as far as the form but only as far as life. If it went as far as the form we would develop a third set of teeth because now human beings are guided by external circumstances. In the external circumstances the situation is such that human beings once again incorporate the extra-human element. When they were guided by the model, they were completely determined by the human being. As long as human beings are guided by the model, they are determined by something hereditary. But that is also what contains the element which has withered. Since the separation from the sun it has been severed from the roots of its existence, has withered, wasted away. That is why the largest number of pathological forces lie in the hereditary forces so that it is indeed the case that human beings incorporate a great deal of the inner causes of disease by their determination through the model. But they incorporate little before puberty because they are guided by the external world; climate and so on, all the things that are present in the external air, are less harmful. Human beings are healthy between the age of seven and 14, but then the period starts again in which they become more susceptible to illness. The image of the human being must be kept in mind while observing all these circumstances. If you have the image of the human being in mind, then you are meditating properly. Then you will be able to combine the things you can learn with what you meditate. Then what you learn does not remain theory but becomes practical experience because you reveal the power which allows you to perceive it. That is the thing which is so much needed today. We simply cannot achieve anything in medicine if we believe that there is a linear progression in development. Human beings are actually composed of broken off developmental streams which run for seven-year periods and a later stream will always connect again with an earlier one. There is no one-sided continuity but other circumstances always intervene. We only find such continuity, in which the previous thing is always the cause of the following one, in the mineral realm, less so in the plant realm and least of all in the human realm.

Start by thinking properly about the plant realm. What do people do today when they think properly about the plants? [See Plate 11] Here we have the soil. Now people imagine that the seed is laid here and the plant starts growing. They are naive enough to think that, well, hydrogen is a very simple molecule, it only consists of two atoms.[31] They dream up all kinds of things. Alcohol is already a more complex molecule. Here carbon is combined with hydrogen and oxygen, giving us something more complex. So then we get the most complex substances with the most complex molecules. There was a time in the 1880s and 1890s when dissertations had the most complex titles extending over two or three lines. Here the molecule is extremely complex. But now it gets even more complex. It becomes a seed, a very complex compound. Then the plant grows out of the seed.

That is nonsense. Seed development works by earthly matter tearing itself out of any kind of structure in the seed and passing over into chaos, becoming chaotic, so that it no longer comprises any material forces. Then those things which work from out of the cosmos can wholly apply themselves if no earthly structure is present any longer. The seed declares its readiness to model the cosmic, the cosmic structure in miniature so that nothingness asserts itself with regard to the earthly in seed development and the cosmic can work into such nothingness. Dr Kolisko[32] could tell you a thing or two to confirm this. For the studies on spleen function[33] we had to take rabbits and remove the spleen from them. The rabbits felt quite well despite that. Indeed, they didn't die from the operation but quite a while later from a cold. It was indeed possible to observe how the rabbits managed without a spleen. When one of the rabbits died, it was possible to look at what happened with regard to the spleen. And, lo and behold, the spleen had been replaced by an actual spherical piece of tissue. What happened? We removed the physical spleen from the rabbit. [See Plate 11 top right] By doing that, we artificially drove the physical substance into chaos and made it accessible to the cosmic forces, allowing something to be created which was similar to seed development. Something was created which at a very primitive level was similar to seed development: that is a reflection of the cosmos. Thus something important was confirmed by this wholly innocent vivisection, because spiritual-scientific observation shows that it is so. [See Plate 11 bottom right]

Take a quartz crystal. It is certainly a physical object. And why is it a physical object? It is an object which pedantically holds on to its shape—the quartz crystal. The quartz has its form through inner strength. And if you smash it with a hammer, the individual parts still maintain their propensity to be pyramids complete in themselves and still hexagonal. This propensity exists. You can remove this propensity from the quartz with as little success as you can remove the pedantry from a pedant. You could also atomize a pedant but he would still be pedantic. You cannot force quartz into a situation in which the cosmos could do something with its forces. That is why it is not alive. If quartz were pulverized to such an extent that the parts no longer had the propensity to be guided by its own forces in each individual part, something cosmic which is alive would grow out of the quartz. That is what happens in the development of the seed. In the latter case matter is expelled to such an extent that the cosmos with its etheric forces can intervene. We have to look at the world as a continuous getting into and emerging from chaos. What is in quartz also once emerged from the cosmos but it has remained and become ahrimanic. It no longer exposes itself to the cosmic forces. As soon as we enter life we always have to keep going through chaos.

That gives you another point of reference for meditating medically. The starting point is that you visualize the fully developed plant as it grows from leaf to leaf and so on. Then you come to the seed development in the fruit and you imagine that it grows very dark, very black, whereas otherwise you imagine the seed plant to be bright. Then the brightness returns in that it is seized again from the outside. So the life of the plant once again allows you to create an imaginative picture; if you are aware that this is the plant, then that is something imaginatively meditative. You must not be intellectual but must remain in the concretely imaginative. The intellectual only exists to put what we know into thought. [See Plate 11]

You could write down the word 'humankind', for example. Well, that is formed from a perception. All right. When you hear the word 'humankind' you are reminded of humankind. But if you now come along and say you like the I so you'll put it at the beginning and the D, you'll put that here, and the H and so on, you can reassemble the word in a different way but it won't actually change anything in a way that you can do anything with it. But that is what people do with concepts all the time. A concept is only an intellectual way of expressing a perception. People separate and combine concepts and think in their thinking. People do the same thing with their external observations. They impose thinking on observation and so people today live outside reality. We can do that as long as we are working with the kind of science which is outside reality such as geometry and arithmetic. But if we want to do medicine we cannot be outside reality because then we are also outside reality in the way we practise medicine.

LECTURE 10

DORNACH, 22 APRIL 1924

My dear friends,

I would like it if today you would really tell me what worries you so that we can hold our discussion with that in mind.

Helene von Grunelius:[34] One question which is of great concern to all of us is how we should cope with all the meditations we have. At what time should we do them? Should we do them in a proper rhythm? How should we do them? Should we do all the ones we were given at Christmas at the same time? Until now at least, it appears that most of us have felt crushed, as it were, by all the meditation material and do not yet know how to live with it properly.

Well you see, with regard to all these things it really is a matter of not giving strict instructions in such a way because that would be intervening too much in human freedom. And if we look at these things in the right way, the soul should not be crushed by them. The meditations which were given here at Christmas were always given in such a way that the direction in which they move the soul was also stated. That was stated with all the meditations such as these. That of course also included meditations such as are now given in the First Class.[35] All these meditations are different from someone coming and asking for a meditation which has a personal effect. If someone wants a meditation which has a personal effect he or she must of course be told whether the meditation concerned should be done in the morning or evening, how such a meditation should be handled in other respects and those kinds of things. These are meditations intended to act on the esoteric life of the person in accordance with his or her abilities and karma. By themselves they then lead to the individual not remaining alone but developing the impulse to recognize all those others who are striving in the same direction. We have to consider such meditations as personal meditations.

Anything else that is given—unless it is stipulated that it would be good for such a meditation to be undertaken at a particular time or under particular circumstances with specific accompanying effects, which has not happened yet—all such meditations which are given like the meditation from the esoteric lesson at Christmas are given in such a way that we observe very precisely the effect achieved by the meditation. And then it is a matter of using the circumstances of one's life, that is the specific situation of our life, to do such meditations. You see, such meditations are simply done when we find the time for them. The more frequently, the better. They will always have the corresponding effect. With such meditations in particular it should always be a matter of striving for personal development. Coming together should then be sought on the basis of what arises for the spirit—and it will be found, so that really the most depressing thing would be if specific instructions were given as to the way that these meditations should be done individually or, as you say, by a whole group at the same time. That would also lead to the meditation losing something which it should really have. You see, it detracts from every meditation if we start from the obligation that we have to do it. You have to be very clear about that. It detracts from every meditation if we start from the obligation that it has to be done. That is why it is so necessary with a personal meditation that such a personal meditation is gradually transformed into something in human beings which they experience in their soul as a thirst for the meditation. And the people who are the most correct in doing the morning and evening meditations they have to do in the most correct way are the ones who have a thirst for the meditation in the same way that people eat when they are hungry. If the meditation becomes something without which we cannot exist, of which we feel with regard to the soul that it belongs to the whole life of the soul, then the meditation is experienced in the right way.

With the other meditations it is a case of really inwardly wanting to become a physician, of telling ourselves this is the path and I will use the meditation as frequently as I can. I am aware that when I do this one or that one it has this or that purpose. The urge must therefore always be there from the free inner volition of the human being to undertake such a meditation. And it is actually unimaginable that this would make one despondent. Because why should the thing for which one is inwardly thirsting make one despondent? If that happens it has already passed over into a kind of obligation and that it should never be, it should never be an obligation. Particularly when we are talking about becoming a physician, we should consider the following in the most profound meaning of the words. Becoming a physician should never be seen in the way it is seen today, as entering a profession. But we should become a physician through an inner calling, the inner devotion to healing and so on. And when we feel this general urge to heal, then this meditation will show us the way and we will be guided to our goal. There are probably few professions other than the medical profession in which it is as damaging to see the work as an external obligation. Love of humanity and a real, natural finding one's way into being a physician are integral parts of the medical profession. Now, if it is not of any great benefit for real healing in medicine today, in medical studies today, if people want to become a physician because they cannot think of anything better and it seemed the best option to them at the time, if that is not particularly desirable it is even less desirable if someone wants to become a physician artificially through meditating if he or she does not feel this thirst of which I have spoken. Because the ancient means, the esoteric means to make progress provide support if the intention is right; they support infinitely more than any outer decision whereas they cause much more damage than the outer circumstances of life if they do not arise from the right soul mood. But now you also have to understand in the right way what I refer to as soul mood here. Normally people do not take what we call karma very seriously. We must, of course, have a certain vocation, let us say, preordained for us in that karma puts us in a particular place; and we must be clear that following an obligation is damaging, but following karma is something that certainly lies in human development. Karma has put all of you in a place where you can work in medicine.

Now you just have to look deeply enough inside yourself and you will find that you really feel that thirst. And you will find the moments, the hours in which you want to do such meditations.

If you sincerely take up such a serious profession, then something must not happen which has happened frequently particularly since the Christmas Conference. It is not related directly to being a physician or to medicine but greatly to general human characteristics in so far as they exist in the general anthroposophical movement—so it is also of importance for you. I will indeed mention it in another place but because it applies to you with particular intensity, I will also say it here. It was said at the Christmas Conference[36] that a new spirit should enter the anthroposophical movement, that inward work should take place. Now some people drew a rather peculiar conclusion from that. There are people who occupy certain positions within the anthroposophical movement, they hold their offices. And now there are these people, who hold their offices, who write: yes, now a new spirit—I fully understand that—will enter the anthroposophical movement. I fully place myself at the service of this new spirit, I do not want to remain in my old office and want to make myself fully available. That will not lead anywhere. It will only lead somewhere if the people concerned know that they have to develop as human beings in the place in which they find themselves, also with regard to the powers they use. And that of course applies particularly to you, who have started out in the medical profession. You have to see it as karma and be clear that you will do much work in the future and, secondly, that the thirst of which I have spoken to you—to approach the real readiness to be a physician by way of meditating—can always be found in the human mind.

That is what I wanted to say about the use of meditation. It should work in such a way that the one illuminates and supports the other, that the one is illuminated by the other. It can quite easily happen that a meditation you did had a strong effect; now you have to do another meditation in order to illuminate this effect to an even greater extent. You might do one meditation once or twice, another one 12 times. That is something that will emerge if you properly take to heart what has been given as a meditation, experience it inwardly and also take to heart what was said with regard to the goal of the meditation. We have to use this opportunity to expand on certain things which were touched on at Christmas.

Helene von Grunelius: It was not that I thought that meditation should be done at certain times; but I nevertheless felt a certain despondency because I took it as an obligation to do this meditation and sometimes did not have the proper freshness to experience it as a need. Now this might be, at least in my case, because until now I simply did not have the attitude which one has to have as a physician, namely the will to heal. I believe that some of us were in this position. We did not become physicians in order to heal, at least some of us, but because of the great interest we had to study the human being—in sickness and in health— and really to approach medicine wholly from the cognitive side. The will to heal was something quite new to me at Christmas and so because of present work I was initially very unhappy because I had a lot to do and was too tired at the beginning to do meditations. Now through this work I began to have more contact with patients so that now I have an idea of the will to heal; and so I think that now I will be better able to do the meditations because then this will arise from a real desire and the meditation will then really be seen as a path to achieve the goal. Precisely such devotion to human destiny, such empathy which we feel with everything as a physician, and the will to heal, that is something which caused many of us difficulties until recently because we were not made aware of it through our studies which tend to approach medicine from the cognitive side.

You have to consider the following. If you separate these two things in the medical field, the cognitive side and the will to heal, you are basically in reality expressing a contradiction. It is important to be clear about what is the case here. You see, we have to talk about the necessity of knowing the human being in a great variety of fields. In education, for example, we have to talk very much about starting from a knowledge of the human being. The same thing happens with us. We also have to talk about a knowledge of the human being in other fields when we look at the reality. A knowledge of the human being is necessary for everyone who wants to get beyond an unskilled approach. Everyone needs to have an understanding of the human being. That such knowledge of the human being is not being sought in the various fields is a consequence of the error which has become widespread in modern culture. You see, knowledge of the human being is indeed being sought today in a certain sense even if it never happens because it can really only be found through anthroposophy. It is being sought by theologians, I mean the outside theologians. The outside educators are also looking for it. Such knowledge of the human being is being sought by a wide variety of people. The only people who are not looking for it are the lawyers because jurisprudence is not something today of which we can say that it connects with the world in reality.

Now you see, the key thing is that a knowledge of the human being must be specialized somewhat in the various fields of life. The physician requires a somewhat different knowledge of the human being from the educator; only somewhat different. It would be necessary for education to be pervaded as much as possible by medicine, and medicine in turn to be pervaded as much as possible by education. Those threads should indeed be tied, the interchange between the one and the other activity based on a knowledge of the human being. If we now look at a knowledge of the human being in concrete terms, we have to ask ourselves the following. You see, when you say 'recognizing a person's pathological state'—that is a preconception which arises from materialism. It is a materialist preconception. What does 'recognizing the pathological state of a person' mean in concrete terms? How do I recognize the disease which is localized, say, in the liver, the spleen, the lung, the heart? How do I recognize it? When I know the healing process which might underlie the disease in order to overcome it. In reality the pathological process is the question and we stop at the question if we only seek to recognize the pathological process. The answer is the healing process. We know nothing about a pathological process if we do not know how to heal it. Such knowledge consists in the understanding as to how the pathological process can be rectified so that there can be no medical studies without the will to heal. Recognizing pathological states means nothing. If we tried to understand the human being by practising pathology without immediately moving on to therapy, that would be equivalent to describing a diseased organ. But such a description is of no value, it does not have the least value. Because with regard to the mere description, with regard to abstract knowledge, with regard to what is now considered to be a knowledge of nature, it is quite irrelevant whether we are dealing with a healthy or diseased liver. It is not possible to distinguish scientifically between a healthy and a diseased liver, or we can do so at most through the circumstance that a healthy liver occurs more frequently than a diseased one. But that is an external circumstance. If we want to recognize a diseased liver we have to think about what can heal the diseased liver. And then, you see, it is about the following.

What forms the basis of healing? That I know the substances and forces I have to apply to the human being so that the disease process is transformed into a healthy process. Such knowledge is provided when I know, let us say for example, that Equisetum assumes the activity of the kidney in the human being, the human organism. So if the activity of the kidney is insufficiently undertaken by the astral body, I have Equisetum do it. I support the astral body with *Equisetum arvense*. But that only provides an answer as to the actual situation which exists. The same process which outwardly produces Equisetum also occurs in the human kidney and I have to look at the Equisetum process in connection with the human kidney; but then I have already moved over to healing. So it can never be a matter of practising pathology in a merely abstract sense because in reality that is nothing. The diseased state should really only be looked at by a person in the context of knowing that a healing medicine works in this or that way. The feeling we have towards knowledge should push us in all fields of life towards reality, not towards formal understanding. That is how it was when all knowledge was mystery knowledge. Knowledge had to be withheld from those who simply wanted to know and it was only given to those who had the will to turn such knowledge into reality.

Does that answer your question?

Helene von Grunelius: Perhaps I was a bit extreme when I only spoke about health and illness. I actually still include the way in which people should be healed in the cognitive aspect. I am referring to something else. That, even when we know how a person can be healed, we may not have the will to heal him or her. Until now I did not have the impulse to understand and experience the human being—how to heal—only in order to heal a person. I did not have this impulse, the impulse to make all of my work, my studies and everything I assimilate as knowledge inwardly infused with this: I have to be able to heal a person.

That is hypertrophy of insight.

Helene von Grunelius: But that is how it is with me and it is a fact which I wanted to put because it exists and it might appear very peculiar—

You see, it is a good thing—you will think this terribly trivial and simple—it is a good thing that clocks cannot do that because otherwise there would be clocks which are properly wound up in accordance with all the skills of the clockmaker's art but which would not want to work. Human beings can develop this or that by letting their will hypertrophy in one direction or another, but that is then something which does not lie in the healthy development of human nature. Knowledge about healing should not actually exist without the will to heal and you should really be speaking about something completely different today. You should not be speaking about that but you should be saying: 'I have only been studying medicine for a short time, now I am filled with an irrepressible will to heal. I have to restrain myself to prevent this will, which comes from knowledge, from bursting out so that I want to start to heal all the healthy people.' I do not say that as a joke. It should really be the voice of restraint which is heard. It should not be possible at all to say: 'I have striven for knowledge of healing but not for the will to heal.' Because knowledge which is real cannot be separated from the will, that is quite impossible.

Another participant: I think that what Miss von Grunelius has said is something, a state, which tends actually to be brought out by the courses as they are taught at university. It seems to me that this is a result which we find as the end result after ten or 12 semesters of study. The whole mindset of medical science is directed at the cognitive side without leading over into the therapeutic aspect. We learn things in the lecture theatres, in the clinical semesters, and throughout the lecture all we hear about is diagnosis; and right at the end, when the hospital bed has already been wheeled out and the professor does not know how to fill the time until the next patient arrives, a few words are dropped in about therapy which are totally useless. A lecturer also said that once. It was on a gynaecology course and the senior physician spoke about the work of the physician in practice: 'Have you not noticed, gentlemen, that basically so little has been said about therapy? You will only notice that once you are engaged in practise. That is what happened to me: I had a head full of facts and that is when I noticed that I had never heard any reference to that ...' He also described how there are only five minutes of talk about therapy and 40 minutes about diagnosis. And no physician had noticed that they had heard nothing about therapy throughout their studies. That also leads me to a question. As a young person who as a physician sought something different in academic medicine, conflicts arise in me as a result of this basic approach of science today. This utterly superficial attitude which comes to expression in all kinds of ways means that things often arise in diagnosis which are abhorrent to the soul and appear outrageous. So I would like to explain that with an example. A patient once came to me with the question whether I could help her. She suffered from a recurring inflammation of the frontal sinuses and she had frequently visited a specialist. A perforation was made from the nose, and so on. And she said she could no longer bear it, she felt too physically interpreted and she could no longer go along with that, could I not help her in another way. This attitude, which the patient experienced in such a sensitive way, is one which we encounter everywhere, which does no more than fumble and search about superficially, leading to nothing—an attitude which might be described as cynical. The result can also only ever remain superficial and will not lead to what is actually happening. So I have often asked myself: is it actually good, or necessary at all, to respond to such an extent to these methods in the form they are given, in the form they have to be gone through in our studies, and which become monstrous in the gynaecological methods of examination which stand in no relationship to what is actually achieved at the end? Is it necessary to go through all these methods? I have the feeling that what is present as the healing instinct in a person is completely suppressed by having to go through all of that. Let me tell what an old colleague said to me. He was not speaking about a physician but a rural healer in the Bavarian mountains. He did all kinds of orthopaedic things with consummate ease so that he became famous. An orthopaedist in Munich heard about his skill, went to see him and told him he should come to his hospital. The man saw all the equipment in the hospital and the professor said to him that he should show him how he did it. The rural healer looked at everything and from that day onwards he could no longer heal. Should we go along with what academic medicine presents to us in the way of methods, scientific methods? Or should we as far as possible not go along with that?

Looked at from this side, the question is exceptionally important. You are, of course, right and I did not want to speak about the personal circumstances of Miss von Grunelius but I just wanted to characterize something which exists as an attitude of necessity as a result of studies today. In proper medical studies it would not occur to anyone to want to know about a person's pathological process or about healing processes without the will to heal. That would not be absent from proper medical studies; it is only absent because of the way that medical studies are set up today. On the one hand we have to say that actually most of what medical students have to study in their semesters has nothing what-soever to do with healing and therefore basically only represents a burden on the human soul with impossible things. You see, medical studies today are rather like asking a sculptor, let us say, first to get to know mainly the scientific characteristics of marble and wood. That is not something he really needs to concern himself with. Much of what is written in textbooks today or what happens in hospitals has nothing to do with medicine. In the instant when you move from a physical description—which the lady experienced when she felt too physically interpreted—to the etheric body, most of the things written in the medical books lose their meaning because in that instant when you move over to the etheric body you obtain a quite different perspective of the organs. In the instant when you move from the physical body to the etheric body intellectual knowledge is no longer sufficient in any way. You will learn a lot more if you learn to sculpt, learn the skills, the spatial sense which a sculptor needs. To understand the astral body you will learn a lot more if you can use musical elements. You will learn an incredible amount about the way the human organism is formed, how this forming process develops out of the astral body. When human beings pass over into activity, they are actually constructed like a musical scale. In the one direction, the prime starts here at the back, changes into the second, changes into the third in the forearm; where there are two thirds the human being also has two bones, and in that way you will learn quite different things from what is used today for a true understanding of the human being. And quite a different course would be required for aspiring physicians than exists today. Today's course has come about precisely because of what has come out now through Miss von Grunelius—that therapy has become nihilistic. Something nihilistic has been introduced not just by the school of Viennese physicians but everywhere. And I have to say that among the physicians, professors and lecturers who represent scientific subjects there were at least serious people who were scientific because of their lack of vision. There was at least a certain seriousness. But when we get to those who lecture on pharmacology, the seriousness stops. There the lecturer himself has stopped believing in what he is lecturing about. Where the serious attitude should start in the course, where the therapeutic part starts, that is where the seriousness stops. Where is the will to heal supposed to come from? From the medical course if it is structured similarly to the way I sketched out following the Christmas course. And that is of course something quite different from what happens today, because that does not lead to pharmacological skills. General practitioners generally have to acquire certain knowledge with great difficulty after they leave university. That is not always so easy because all those things are not just useless but often damaging. They cannot see the actual disease process because they have all kinds of things in their heads, in their memory, and cannot see the actual disease process. That is the one side.

On the other hand, the other side is this. You are a group of young physicians here. Not only do you want spiritually to become proper physicians, which would of course be achieved best if you were told, 'Leave your medical studies, you will not find a medical faculty today where you can study medicine. Come here and learn what you need to learn.' That is what we could say quite radically. But what would the young physician do? The world would reject you because it would not recognize you as a physician. There is no alternative for young physicians other than to go through the whole process in order then to be healed by what you can learn about medicine at the Goetheanum. But you have to put yourself through the regular, proper course even if you are reluctant to do so; there is no alternative. It is a necessity. That is the other side. But once there are quite a number of those who are familiar with such studies and as a result know how things should not be—after all, magnetopaths and lay practitioners also complain about the universities, but that is not worth anything—they will learn from that experience and they will be the proper pioneers so that we can have sensible medical studies in the world. That is what you should be striving for, to try as far as possible to get the public to see what is happening.

You see, basically the situation is this. As you know, you are not the only ones to say the things you have said. There are many physicians who speak like that—but those who speak like that need exactly what is offered here in addition. Why? You can, of course, criticize official medicine if you are reasonable people and become physicians and have gone through a university course. You have gone through it and know what we do not have. But it can only become effective if there is something to put in its place. Only then will the whole thing become effective. That is the other side, of course. That is why you should not take all the things I have said here to mean that I want to stop any of the young physicians from completing their studies. As bad as it is, we still have to bite the bullet today. Things will only gradually improve if we can talk from a basis of what should not be.

You see, there is still quite a lot to do in that respect. I think I have already told you this story. I was once asked to talk about medical matters to a group of physicians in Zurich and the professor of gynaecology had come along. Now I could see that he had come with the inner attitude: 'Let's hear this rubbish so that at least we can criticize and say we were there.' He really came ready for a joke to listen to this rubbish. But then he acted more and more strangely and listened in a strange way. He found it most unpleasant that it was not rubbish, that it was not something of which he could say it was pure nonsense. I found that particularly amusing. I addressed him: 'Professor, you had a strange impression.' He responded: 'Well, you can't talk about that, it is simply a different perspective.' It is indeed progress if we reach the stage where people think that it is a different perspective. What is it that has appeared alongside a scientific medicine which even so still towers above what has been achieved by lay medicine? I know that the lay practitioners have achieved important progress; but that is not relevant. A small boy found a way to automate the way the valves open and close in a steam engine because he was bored. But that does not mean he was a mechanical engineer because he found a way to do that. The people who stand here today and complain mainly about scientific medicine are not really entitled to do so and they refer to something of which they have no knowledge. We still have to get to the point where the anthroposophical aspect of medicine is not confused with the other things that exist. Significant progress will have been made once we have achieved a situation in which the matter is taken seriously because the people who represent it show that they take it seriously.

It is something I would particularly like to entrust to you young friends, to make everything that you receive as esoteric material reach the point where you can work in the world, so that a proper will to heal really does develop. It cannot be a matter of locking yourself away egotistically in your own little world but you must work to bring progress to medicine and so on, just as the teachers are working to bring progress to education.

It is not possible for me to set out in detail how most of the things which medical courses do today are actually unnecessary for an understanding of the reciprocal relationship which exists in the healthy and sick human being. But if you study what I have offered in the various courses and cycles you will undoubtedly find it. It is as if a child were born and we were faced with the question as to how it was to be fed and asked ourselves: is it possible to feed the child before having taught him or her an opinion about the different foods? That is the case with many things. I do not mean physically, but spiritually, that we have the intuition to understand the process. It is often a lot more necessary in diagnosis to go back to initial causes, which can lie in a certain period far in the past of the patient, instead of going for the common diagnosis.

You see, recognizing the state of the ill or healthy organism at the moment in which the patient presents himself is what is taught today; there are methods for that. But the way of thinking which allows us to say to the patient you experienced this or that 50 years ago and that is the original cause of your illness—people do not have that; they rely on what the patient tells them and that can be unreliable. This initial cause in particular is the external cause which comes from the outside. A man was presented to me by a physician in Oslo.[37] He was 60 years old. He had all kinds of rashes which were easy to diagnose. But none of the treatment helped. So the physician brought him to me—I mention one example among hundreds—and it was clear above all that if we were to do something we would have to know how the whole thing started. It was not very difficult. I soon discovered that the man had gone through a severe poisoning process 30 or 35 years ago. That is what was inside him. I told him he should recall what had happened to him 35 years ago. He told me: 'No one has yet asked me about that. I was at school. A chemical laboratory was next to our classroom where I saw a glass with liquid. I was thirsty and drank it. I was terribly poisoned because it was hydrochloric acid.' Knowing that is incredibly important. It stands out from the current situation. So it can be important to know in, let us say, some hysterical nervous states whether the person concerned has gone through the shock of almost drowning. We have to go into these things. But we go into these things as a matter of course if we feel empathy for the person whom we want to heal. Everything medical has to start with feeling empathy for a person. If we do not feel such empathy we will forget important things. That is what we should consider in this respect.

Do all of you intend to be here tomorrow still? Then we will continue our considerations tomorrow. But I would like to give you—without going into it further now, but I will explain it tomorrow—a number of lines for further contemplation which can become a kind of central meditation in the direction that was touched on here yesterday. In that way you will get to understand what has been built into the human being from the cosmos, from the surroundings of the earth and by the forces of the earth if you keep directing your attention to that. If you ask about the design of the eye, 'How is this configured out of the cosmos?,'

with the lung, 'How is it configured out of the forces of the periphery,
out of planetary movement, also in the elements of air and water?,' and,
'How does the principle which configures metabolic organs in human
beings relate to the earthly principle?,' if you ask these questions con-
sistently everywhere and meditate as follows, then you will learn to see
into the human being.

> See how things come together in the cosmos
> You sense how the human being is configured.

—that in connection with the moon.

> See what moves you in the air

—for example in the respiration or blood circulation—

> You experience the human being ensouled.

—that is in connection with the sun.

> See what is transformed on the earth,

—especially also what brings death to human beings—

> You grasp how the human being is filled with spirit.

—that in connection with Saturn.

> See how things come together in the cosmos,
> You sense how the human being is configured.　　　　　☾
>
> See what moves you in the air
> You experience the human being ensouled.　　　　　☉
>
> See what is transformed on the earth,
> You grasp how the human being is filled with spirit.　　♄

LECTURE 11

DORNACH, 23 APRIL 1924

M<small>Y</small> dear friends,
I would like to begin by saying a few words about the verse which I
wrote on the blackboard at the end of yesterday's session. It starts with
the words: [See Plate 12]

> See how things come together in the cosmos
> You sense how the human being is configured.   ☾

And I pointed out that the moon symbol has been placed next to it.
Now if we want to understand human beings thoroughly, particularly
with regard to treating them medically, we must be quite clear that we
cannot just look at what links human beings with the earth; because
that, as we saw in the first session, really only concerns the first few years
of childhood up to the change of teeth—and no more thereafter. Then
those forces come into play which actually organize human beings,
organize them away from the earth. They have their etheric body for
that and the etheric body is significantly different from the physical
body. The physical body is heavy, the etheric body is not heavy. The
physical body strives towards the earth, the etheric body in all directions
out into the widths of the cosmos. You will certainly encompass the
whole of the cosmos when you consider the human physical and the
etheric body. The physical body is intimately connected with the earth,
the etheric body is in intimate connection with everything that can be
perceived in the environment surrounding the earth; so you can think of
all the forces which act on your physical body as forces which draw the

human being to the earth and all the forces which act on the etheric body as those which draw the human being away from the earth. They are there and they act in the human being, and so we cannot look at human beings such that we say they assimilate some substance and first it was outside and then it is inside. That is not how it is. Due to the fact that these centrifugal forces are active in human beings, the substance immediately becomes part of the whole universe, the whole visible universe.

Then, if we look at the astral part of the human being, you have to imagine that it actually arises outside space; it only appears to work in space.

And when you get to the I you can no longer make any drawing at all. It works neither from above nor below; it does not work at all in a way such that one could make a drawing of it but it works only through the progression of time, the continuity of time. What emanates from the human I-organization cannot basically be drawn but we must be clear that it is real in every respect; but it radiates neither in nor out in the way it works but works purely qualitatively.

When you look into the etheric worlds, we can say that it is as if we were constantly losing ourselves with our etheric body in the etheric worlds. [See Plate 13] The astral always radiates towards us; it is not spatial either but it acts as if it was coming towards us from the reaches of the cosmos. Now you see, let us assume that in nutrition we are dealing with vegetable protein. Vegetable protein is firstly heavy and secondly, being protein, it also strives towards the cosmos. When you introduce vegetable protein into the human organism then the other two forces immediately arrive through this vegetable protein, the forces which work in from all sides and those which really work non-spatially on the protein as forces of the I-organization. Now assume that all the things which could act on human beings in this way would, grotesque as this may sound, only be able to turn them into round, spherical bodies. You find the shape which arises through the interaction of these forces—the forces radiating out from the earth and those radiating in— in a bird's egg. That is the form which these forces take. But how does it happen that it is not just the shape of the egg which emerges from a bird's egg but a shape with a specific configuration? Well, you see, if there was only what I have drawn here [R.S. draws] then the egg would develop no further than an egg shape. [See Plate 13] The bird would be completed once the egg is there. But it is the case that a bird has a very specific configuration and—what I am about to say about birds also applies to humans—this arises in the first place because the moon orbits the earth. The moon is in orbit. But if we only had the moon orbiting, there still would be no bird. What would happen is that the eggshell would soften and drop off and a spherical entity would develop, a spherical entity consisting essentially of protein. It is not, however, the case that the only thing which the moon does is to orbit the earth; there are many different constellations in space and the moon travels past these constellations, modifying the forces coming from them. Think, therefore, that the moon travels past the Pleiades here. The egg is subject to the forces which stream in from the Pleiades but which are modified by the moon partially covering, that is, modifying them. So a force streams in from the Pleiades which is modified by the moon positioned before them and exercising its influence; as a result the head of the bird develops on the one hand, if I draw it diagrammatically, from the egg. So we can say that the head of the bird is formed from out of the cosmos in the interaction between the moon, a satellite, and the fixed stars which exercise a particular influence because of their arrangement in the Pleiades. Now the moon moves on and, let us say, stands in opposition to its earlier configuration facing Libra. The forces of Libra are modified in turn because of the moon positioned there. We have a different constellation of forces and the moon, which was a full moon here in front of the Pleiades, has in the meantime changed into new moon. The moon in connection with the constellation of Libra has a different effect from when it acts from the Pleiades and the effect on the egg is to create the tail. The other things lie in between so that if you wish to study the shape of the bird you have to study how the moon passes in front of what is spread out cosmically in space. What can anyone say about the development of human beings, or any living thing, if they stop at earthly circumstances? They can only say: certainly the eagle has a certain shape, the vulture has a certain shape, the kangaroo has a certain shape, and so on. Why do they have that shape? If you remain stuck in the terrestrial, like science does, there is only one answer: the animal has inherited its shape from its parents. That is rather like saying there is poverty because people are poor. But it fails to explain anything. You have to keep going further up the chain. The parents have it from their parents and finally you end up where you started. If we want to understand the configuration, we have to go to the cosmic forces, the constellations.

But even that is not the end of it. If only those things existed which I have mentioned, there would certainly be wonderfully formed beings but they would really all be jellyfish, as humans indeed were in past periods of the earth. In the Atlantean period they were a kind of jellyfish. That was so because they were only able to assimilate matter, substance, which was in a malleable, fluid state in order to build their physical bodies. They can integrate potassium, sodium and the other substances because the moon not only travels past Libra, Aries, Taurus but because the other planets in our solar system travel past and they incorporate those things in us which, for example, ensure that we really do get our human shape. So the moon for example—I described a bird to you—also has simultaneously incorporated—I have only drawn the moon, sun and Saturn—those things which also come from the relative position of Mercury to the planets and the relative position of Venus to the planets with regard to the formation of the human head. If they did not act together with the moon in its relative positions we would all be born with hydrocephalus. That is how we have the organic metal characteristics incorporated in us, that the relative positions of Mercury and Venus work together with the relative positions of the moon. And we would suffer dreadfully from rickets, not just be bow legged but have legs that bend elastically and our arms would be jellyfish-like, if on the other hand those planets did not act together in relation to the moon which are directed more at Saturn and if Saturn itself did not work together with Jupiter and Mars. The sun causes the rhythmical balance between these two parties.

So these first two lines of the verse are intended to lead you to understand how the human being is formed out of the cosmos. And we will not make any progress until astronomy is reintroduced into our medical science—but astronomy in the sense I have explained it now. In fact most of the things which people say tend not to have any great meaning. They juggle, don't they, between earthly circumstances and heredity by ascribing the phenomena in human beings either to one or the other. But if you look at it in detail you get nowhere because it has been forgotten that the way in which human beings develop must be derived from what is provided by a knowledge of the starry sky—but seen qualitatively in its inner nature. But the most important thing with regard to the human form is the moon. That has to be involved everywhere while the others modify its influence. The most important thing with regard to the human form is the moon.

The second line says: [See Plate 12]

> See what moves you in the air
> You experience the human being ensouled. ☉

You see, everything at work in the human etheric body forms the human being. But human beings would become living robots, even if they had our form today, if the only thing acting on them were what I have described so far. But that is not the only thing that acts on them but the environment also acts, all that is alive and active in the element of the air which surrounds us. And the etheric and the astral from the cosmos are also active in the air. And just as we are formed and shaped externally and spatially under the influence of the moon combined with the heavens, so we include in our form inward ensoulment because the sun works together with the heavens for this just like the moon does for our form. So we can say that when the sun influences the cosmic forces in such a way that it is positioned in front of Leo, then it first works—now we are no longer talking about our own forces, please note—in the surrounding air on what acts on us through our respiration and the blood circulation, and this changes constantly. The air changes as the sun moves on. This action in the surroundings internalizes the form to become ensoulment so that we can truly say the sun constellations in the cosmos have their effect in the surroundings of the earth in the airy element and that provides our ensoulment. So that is the second one.

The third line says: [See Plate 12]

> See what is transformed on the earth,
> You grasp the human being filled with spirit. ♄

This transformation refers to the gradual sinking down of the physical body into the corpse. 'See what is transformed on the earth, You grasp the human being filled with spirit.' But Saturn has to be included. Why? Well, you see, the Saturn forces are not just up there where Saturn is positioned. Saturn is located in space a long distance from the earth and its external action is not particularly great. It does not act a great deal externally on human beings. Its constellations with regard to other stars do not have a particularly strong effect on human beings either. But it has forces which are soaking very strongly into the earth. The Saturn forces soak very strongly into the earth and when we look outwards we do not really find many Saturn forces. But when we look at the earth itself, at what there is from the surface towards the inside of the earth, we see that it is rather like what I might describe as what happens when you see a snail moving along the ground. You have the snail going past, and when you look where it has gone you see a trail of slime which it has left behind. You can see where it has gone. The same thing happens with Saturn. It moves along but leaves traces behind in all the places where it has shone on the earth. These are very, very clear traces. If these traces had not remained in much earlier periods of earth development as forces which inhabit the earth, we would have no lead anywhere in the earth. Lead is created from the original substance, from the Saturn forces at work in the earth itself which have soaked in. The lead forces were created in the earth in more ancient periods, when circumstances were different. Today the lead forces do still have an after-effect in human beings and they have quite a different effect from the other two forces. You see, we would not be people with a mind but beings with a body and soul if the Saturn forces did not exist. That should tell you something, my dear friends. In reality there is nothing without a reason in the cosmos. Ask yourselves: during what period has Saturn had an opportunity to impregnate the earth from all sides with its forces? It has done so in the course of 30 years in which it has orbited it—the sun and thus the earth. These 30 years are also the 30 years which human beings spend from birth until the time when a certain development in their lives has been concluded. When human beings have lived for 30 years on earth, then, where they stand on earth, they are precisely at the point—which might not of course necessarily coincide with the straight line coming from Saturn in the heavens—where Saturn has impregnated the earth; it impregnates the spot for the second time when human beings have reached the age of 30. And so the influence of Saturn on the earth is wholly connected with human beings and that is ultimately why we have a body which has catabolism, as we keep saying. We do not just have anabolic forces in the organism because that would make us pass out; our vitality has to recede in a certain way. The catabolic forces must always be there. Our organism not only develops in a forward direction but its development also recedes and the space for spiritual development lies in this receding development—that is where it goes. Spiritual development does not come out of vitality but as the latter recedes spiritual development finds a space in what has been left empty, metaphorically. That comes from the forces which arise in the earth through the impregnation of the earth with the Saturn forces. That is why I had to put the Saturn symbol with the third verse. [See Plate 12]

However, as people we would be ancient old men and women at the age of 30 because of these Saturn forces. We would have to start walking on crutches at 30. Indeed, Fichte[38] was happy to accept the worth of human beings but only until they were 30. He said that all 30-year-olds should be killed because from then on they were no longer of any use to the world and became weak cripples. What Fichte meant by that would inevitably happen if Saturn were indeed able to unfold its forces on earth. But the Saturn forces are also modified by the Jupiter and Mars forces. As a result we do not catabolize to the same extent up to the age of 30 but only to the degree that we can carry on for a bit beyond then, and it is indeed due to Mars and Jupiter that we are not ancient old people by the age of 30. If we want to understand how human beings can still be human beings at 45 we have to look out into cosmic space. And so the moon, sun and Saturn are the celestial bodies which are nearest to us and furthest from us in the planetary system. The way it is structured today is not organic because up to Saturn[39] it emerged from an earlier single whole whereas Uranus and Neptune came in and became part of it at a later stage. Uranus and Neptune had not been discovered by the ancients, which is why they took Saturn to be the outermost planet. There continues to be good reason for going as far as Saturn. Astrologers still have an awareness of this in that they really only use Uranus and Neptune for those human characteristics which go beyond the personal, for when human beings become inspired or strive to go further than what is personal to the individual, for when we are concerned with things which are no longer connected with personal development. That is the general approach in astrology. Only when human beings become inspired or strive beyond their human nature, let us say, or when their organization expands or catabolizes excessively—everything, then, which goes beyond human nature applies in this respect. They are the planets which behaved like cosmic drifters and were then captured by the planetary system which goes with our earth. The celestial body nearest to us and the celestial body farthest from us regulate what occurs in human beings: the moon with regard to our form; Saturn, through the earth, with regard to our formless spiritual part in that it breaks down our form, always dissolving it in an inward direction. And the sun brings about the rhythm between the two. There you have what we really need to know. On the basis of ancient experience it was possible to know that the forces which correspond to our third line, 'See what is transformed on the earth, You grasp the human being filled with spirit', are the same complex of forces which first came to expression in lead formation. So that we can say that what fissures us as a physical organism so that there is room for the spiritual element must also occur in lead. It is fissuring forces which have created lead. If we introduce lead into the human organism, fissures arise. If we need fissuring because we catabolize too little we must give lead in some form or other. If, in contrast, the opposite is the case, so that human beings cannot create sufficient form, that they become what we might call spongy, then the ancient knowledge must be applied so that the force streaming in from the moon in ancient times when the minerals were formed, the silver substance, should act; in other words, the complex of moon forces is at work in that instance so that the silver forces are the forces which turn sponginess into structure. Silver substance can support the power of the moon.

The whole of the planetary system is connected with those agents which are preferentially used for medicines: Saturn = lead, Jupiter = tin, Mars = iron, sun = gold, Venus = copper, Mercury = mercury and the moon with silver. These concordances are treated in an incredibly superficial way, based, as they are, on the meticulous studies that were undertaken in the ancient mysteries. It is indeed true that things were tested at that time in a much better and more concrete way because these conclusions are based on something that has been well tested. The position of Saturn was examined very closely when the constitution of the whole organism in a person lost independence so that the fissuring forces did not work sufficiently; the vitality, the integrating forces became too strong so that the person became dazed in his or her organic constitution; it does not necessarily have to be the sensorium which becomes dazed. The ancients would see that it happened when Saturn was in a particular position so that Saturn still had a very strong effect on human beings in earlier times. If it was observed that human beings fell into such a state just when Saturn was setting, when it could not unfold its forces in full, then lead was used as a medicine. The information about these things, which can still be found in amateurish books today, is indeed true for the reason that people cannot spoil it because they do not know where it comes from; otherwise people would speculate about it and then we would quite certainly have bad information. It remains correct because people have lost the science from which it originates. It remains through tradition. People cannot spoil this truth through thinking. Even those effects which act on human beings from the earth are in truth the action of Saturn which has simply been retained, drawn in by the earth.

Just consider the magnificent consequences all of this has with regard to human understanding. It is quite impossible to link the moral element with the human being as he or she is seen by science today; the moral element remains adrift somewhere up there in the abstract. That is also why it is particularly in Protestantism, which has lost the connection with the spiritual, with the cosmos, that everything of a moral nature is simply separated off from a cosmic context. All that remains is pure belief. But when you look at reality, human beings are definitely creatures sustained and maintained from out of the cosmos and the moral forces flow in together with their astral nature. Then you have the possibility of thinking of the human being as truly inwardly connected with the moral world. Thus you return once again, if you practise true medicine, to what makes human beings moral entities at all, to the human being who can experience the moral element truly organically and no longer needs to keep it in mind as external commandments.

That is what I wanted to tell you and what I think you can take away with you because it will be able to guide you in many things. You can of course obtain the details in all kinds of places. But the way in which these details behave in the human organism is the thing which you can only obtain from the kind of discussion we have just had. You might be able to read in a medical Vademecum that lead has this or that effect. You will understand why it does that if you have really taken in what we have examined here. It is a feature of all these discussions that, because they are fetched from out of the spiritual world, they demand much less of the memory than what human beings take in physically. What they learn—well, it's like this—they have a certain amount of control over it. But what they obtain in other ways and what implants itself in their memory by itself, that is what you take in by this means. You will notice something particular about it: if you do not keep experiencing it through meditation you will forget it. Spiritual truths have the particular characteristic that they cannot become real remembered truths just as you cannot retain in your organism what you ate a week ago. Ruminants can do so, but only for a short period. In ruminants it is an organic replication, a rudiment in the physical body for what is otherwise only present in the etheric body as memory. But what has to happen with regard to spiritual truths is that they have to be experienced again and again so they then turn into a habit; they are not retained in the memory or pictorially but become habitual. That is the meaning, the comprehensive meaning of meditating—that we appeal to something which basically is only present in early childhood. At that time we do not have any pictorial memory either, that is why young children forget their first experiences. They live in the habitual memory. We have to return to that if we want to deal with spiritual truths in us, otherwise we forget them very quickly.

That is why, because you wanted to receive esoteric material here, I had to call on you to make these things your own inwardly through meditation, otherwise they will be of no use to you. If you meditate, you will develop the delicate receptivity which will enable you—not instinctively now, but through intuition—to feel something similar to what has been preserved in an abstract way in the so-called doctrine of signatures, that is, you will be able to see in the plant or the stone how they can work in the organism. Furthermore, you will not only train your physical body but also your etheric body. And your habitual memory will give you a refined perceptual ability with regard to the content of your physical environment and the ability therefore to look at the world as a person who receives the question from the human organism, the diseased lung, the diseased heart, and the answer from the medicinal plant, the medicinal mineral and so on in the surroundings.

Question: Dr Steiner, many of us are intent on obtaining an orientating, clearest possible overall understanding of the whole situation in which we basically find ourselves. One can feel deep inside oneself that the anthroposophical truths are something quite radical and that an infinite amount depends on their realization. In the newsletter we were sent after the Christmas conference, it struck me how much the meditation given there seems to point towards something generally educational. How can that be realized, which we feel called upon so deeply within ourselves, and how do we obtain a guiding understanding of our own destiny and our tasks in the future? One feels that one can only act in the right way if one learns to understand one's own karma in the greater context and at the same time musters the courage not to want to escape it but to realize it in the right way.

Now I believe I can hear in your question what you want to say. But if I have misunderstood, you will have to rephrase it. The question you have asked touches on something which should be known about today. Because particularly in recent times there has been much discussion in anthroposophical groups of young people, among young people more so than among the old ones, about the end of the Kali Yuga. That is so because it is indeed the case that with the end of the nineteenth century a new age of humanity has started. To begin with, people continue as they did before. If you have a ball and push it with your hand it will roll, and if you take your hand away it will continue rolling. In the same way, what people experienced up to the end of the nineteenth century con-tinues rolling for the time being, even if the forces are no longer behind it, and it can even take on much worse forms than in the period which has finished. But alongside that, alongside the old period, a light-filled period is arising in the world in a concealed way. A period of lightness is shining into the world and it is indeed the case that the first rays of the period of lightness must be caught by anthroposophy. Now you see, I am talking about certain contexts in much more radical terms now than was the case at the Christmas Conference. You will see the same from the lectures which I otherwise give. Those who can still be here this evening will see that certain human situations are indeed touched upon in the lectures. But with such observations it is not yet possible for me to talk in detail in quite concrete terms about those things which would feed a craving for sensationalism. You see, strict laws have to be observed in these things and I do know that a certain desire need not necessarily be driven only by a craving for sensationalism, that it can exist, and that it can be satisfied if each individual person could be told about their previous lives on earth. Things cannot be taken that far. But certain perspectives can be set out, however, which can become important.

Now you see, it is indeed the case that in ordinary human life today, if I may put it like that, we have two types of people. There are these two types of people because at certain periods the spiritual development of humanity on earth was different from other periods and there was a kind of wave movement. But the waves would not only follow one another, but also run side by side. At certain times, for example, the western development of Christianity had become superficial, externalized. People had no possibility of getting to the content from what was offered to them by Christianity. This provoked a reaction among the Cathars. So there were people who lived very much in external things and people who wanted strongly to develop inwardly. Something similar was the case when under the influence of Comenius[40] and earlier still the communities of the Moravian Brethren were founded deep into Hungary and Poland so that people who were striving deeply in their soul for spirituality were always living together in the world with those who were forced into externality through the karma of their culture. That one person belongs to one group and another to the other is connected with previous karmic circumstances. Now a very significant factor for humanity today is the extent to which a person belonged to the one or other of the groups just described in their earlier incarnation. Let us assume that a person is born today who lived within a Christian tradition which was completely externalized; that person will possess quite a different human configuration from a person who, if you like, belonged to the Bohemian or Moravian Brethren. And what is that difference? You see, you only discover the pertinent facts about the end of the Kali Yuga if you look at the concrete circumstances, otherwise it remains a historical construct. The dark age ran until 1899, then the age of light began. Knowing this is not very productive. We have to deal with concrete spiritual things. The people who are born about the turn of the end of the Kali Yuga are such that they have a strong spiritual striving within them. That should not make you presumptuous but you must include that in your living knowledge. These people are to a large extent people who have their origin in the heretics, in those who wanted to follow an inward path. At about the turn of the nineteenth to the twentieth century, people were called down who did not live in the general stream of externalizing Christianity but in such inward looking sects. What is the consequence of that?

You see, when we pass through the time between death and a new birth we study and obtain a very precise knowledge of the human cosmos in a spiritual way, just like here on earth we can study and get to know the world and cosmos outside the human being. The human cosmos is just as big and detailed because human beings contain just as much as the cosmos. We study that with our transformed will forces. We get to know the human being very precisely. Now there is a difference between the two groups of human beings which I have just spoken about. Those who adopted a more outward path were not able to enter the spiritual world properly between death and a new birth. They passed by the particular nature of human beings in the spiritual world without a thought and were reborn. And it was particularly the people born in the second third of the nineteenth century who were of the type who adopted such an external attitude in their previous life. They did not bring any understanding of the human being with them into their life on earth. They behaved towards the human being such that they used the body for eating, drinking, walking, standing and sitting but they were not interested in such an understanding because they had not absorbed such an interest between death and a new birth. Those were the people who were primarily satisfied with materialism because they did not feel the need to acquaint themselves with the human being. The materialist who only ever wants to know about matter knows the least about it. We can say with a clear conscience that all the people sitting here are reborn souls of heretics—except that you should not consider this as a sign of special merit—who experienced a strong urge between death and a new birth to crawl into every part of the human being and thus have unconsciously turned the human being into an enormous riddle for themselves. That comes to expression in the desire to learn more than is offered by materialistic medicine, and there you have the inner justification for the karma of which you have spoken. You must not take these things lightly because if you took them lightly you would misjudge yourself. You would not get close to what you actually want to get close to as a result of certain experiences you had between death and a new birth. And the result of not finding in our earthly life what we have striven for over centuries is not just that people become superficial. We have left the age behind when people who have learnt truths about the human being between death and a new birth can become superficial without any consequences. Young people are not currently in a position in which they could become superficial without consequences because they would ruin themselves inwardly right down as far as the organs. The worst thing is not that people today are materialistic in their thoughts, that they chatter about monism and so on, that is not the worst thing—we could easily get over that. What people talk about is not of such great import, but what then goes back into the feeling and will nature of the human being is active in the organs and people will not be able to sleep properly at all unless they deepen themselves spiritually. That is the key thing. If you leave people today without such deepening, what will be the consequence? The consequence will be that we need hardly look as far ahead as 1940 or 1950 before there will be widespread epidemics of sleeplessness. Such people will no longer be able to support human civilization at all. So your karma does not give you the choice to ignore it as people could still do before the end of the Kali Yuga and [until] now. You do have to

consider in all seriousness what I have told you now about the configuration of your karma. Of course it has to remain a general characterization but you can nevertheless find the general karma useful with
regard to yourself if you put yourself in the position of frequently
reflecting on the special circumstances of your life. You would, to a
greater or lesser extent, be able to put yourself in a position of finding
something of note if you reflected on the particular circumstances of
your life. The youth movement is too theoretical and as a result we hear
too much of the same theories. If you were to go no further than really
observing in yourselves the special things which young people experience today, which are truly different from what the previous generation
experienced, the youth movement would at once take on a completely
different shape. That is what we are striving for with our youth
movement, that it takes concrete shape and does not remain stuck in
abstractions.

Dr Bort:[41] In the discussion we had yesterday, we not only asked ourselves the question, how come that we were guided to come to Dornach
at Christmas in particular, but we told ourselves that we do not know
with our conscious human being why we have come here at all, and that
the opportunity was presented to us to take in such great things which
we cannot comprehend and have not deserved with what we are. On the
basis of that fact in particular it came alive in many of us that a very
specific task lies ahead of us and that for us it is a matter of being
prepared to tackle this karma and this task just in the way it was
presented to us in the topic which was indicated to us in the newsletter.

Well, if you let the—as I believe—serious discussion we have had work
on your soul, you will be able to take something away with you from
this all too short gathering.

LECTURE 12

DORNACH, 24 APRIL 1924

My dear friends,

I thought that we would continue with what we started by supplementing some of the things I talked about yesterday from another angle. Perhaps the questions which you asked and which Dr Wegman discussed with me can be formulated appropriately in that way.

You see, you grow into the medical, the healthcare profession through your general human destiny. You find a particular stream in the healthcare profession today, and you grow into it such that you rightly feel an inner opposition to it in your mind. Now you have to consider that there are often objective reasons for that and they will become clear to you the more you understand that the medical stream today is in a sense really a foreign body in many things which live in European, in Western civilization. We can only truly understand this when we know that our science and many things which have come about in recent spiritual development have arisen because key individuals in the progress of medicine and science were reincarnated from Arabic and Islamic culture. These matters have recently been addressed a lot here at the Goetheanum[42] and are also connected in other respects with what is currently underway in the anthroposophical movement. But they are certainly also of great relevance for physicians. I have already mentioned in various places how we must look at those spiritual centres which flourished in the same period in which spiritual life prevailed in a primitive way, we might say, in Europe under Charlemagne.[43] At the same time a spiritual culture flourished in the East which was held together by Harun al-Rashid.[44] He had many of the wise men of the time, who also included many physicians, at his court. And you will have noticed that, in explaining these things, we are touching on a time in which Christianity had been at work for hundreds of years.

Now, Christianity itself entered the world as something that can only be understood slowly and gradually; and for an external view, not for an inward one, it is very strange how the profound aspects of Christianity have not actually been penetrated by people so far. Christianity entered the world as an objective fact and human capacities, the capacities of comprehension were not strong enough to develop what actually lies in Christianity in all directions. Hence its objective progress is such that Christianity lives everywhere in the subconscious but human beings have completely ruined this Christianity in the last three or four hundred years. Human beings ruined Christianity through what they know, what is seated in the intellect, the consciousness. Furthermore, we now have the dreadfully amateurish institutions which the universities have been turned into in recent times. In earlier periods there were traditionally four faculties: philosophy, theology, jurisprudence and medicine. What has been added since then has really only happened on the basis of the most outward, murky misunderstanding. Because political faculties, economic faculties were created out of a thinking which no longer had any idea of what we are dealing with. The thing which has failed to be understood, an understanding of which has been completely obscured, is that Christ first sent out four figures to proclaim Christianity to the world: the theologian Matthew, the jurist Mark, the physician Luke and the philosopher John. In this context, which is a very profound one, is rooted what will have to develop in the future. These things only exist in embryonic form; they still have to grow and bear fruit. What is deeply rooted in the spiritual life is that the Gospels cannot agree in their wording because the one is written from the perspective of the theologian, the next from the perspective of the philosopher, the third one from the perspective of the jurist and the fourth from the perspective of the physician. That is something which must be understood. And because the Gospel of Luke has in reality not in any way been taken as an inner instruction with regard to the will to heal—the matter has not been understood—it has come about that the Christian will to heal does not really live in our way of thinking today but has immersed itself in spiritual culture through an Arabism which has taken hold of Christianity like a vice.

It is very interesting, isn't it! Christianity which arose in Asia makes its way to Europe and spreads in Europe. But now look at the court of Harun al-Rashid where the old medicine lived; there the ancient mystery knowledge still lived in the understanding of the human being— the tradition still existed there. Now two people lived at that time: Harun al-Rashid himself, who organized the whole thing, this giant cultural academy which grew under his influence; and then there was someone else who in previous times had been an initiate—at that time the initiation was not revealed. Harun al-Rashid returned as Sir Francis Bacon.[45] He renewed the scientific thinking in the West with a way of thinking that was rooted in Arabism. The soul took this path during the time between death and a new birth [Rudolf Steiner draws, see Plate 14] If you studied Bacon you would see how much entered medicine by that route in particular. You would be astonished. On the other hand the second person, the initiate, reincarnated in the soul of John Amos Comenius. We see how a life striving for the spirit was present in Comenius but he did everything in accordance with intellectual ideas. We can also see how another personality, who did not live at the same time as Harun al-Rashid but played a role in the Battle of Jerez, returned as Darwin. Thus all the people active in science, and particularly in medicine, are reincarnations of something which came to Europe in ancient ideas through the grip in which Arabism held Christianity, but with the exclusion of Christianity—not in the further development of Christianity but with the exclusion of Christianity. And so medicine in particular is something which has mostly entered this way whereas the impulse which is contained in the Gospel of Luke with regard to medicine is still such that we have to say that it still needs to be accepted. To achieve this you have to be able to take the kind of things I discussed yesterday about the cosmic understanding of the human being, an understanding of the human being coming from the cosmos, with the greatest possible seriousness; then you will feel yourself placed in the right way in the tasks which arise for you through your karma. Because, you see, the thing is this. Let us look at the kind of medicine that lived at the court of Harun al-Rashid. It certainly contained, on the one hand, the positive aspect of the Hippocratic way of thinking. Those who might have read the first medical course[46] which I gave here will have seen that I immediately discussed there the principle that Hippocrates[47] was the last one to heal on the basis of the ancient mystery medicine. Now when Hippocratic medicine was transplanted to Asia, a strong stream of Mongolian ways of healing which came from north-east Asia entered it. Much flowed into it against which not only the thinking had to rebel in Europe but also the inner organization of human beings themselves had to rebel, for the inner human organization is not suited to what entered medical thinking there as Mongolian and Tartar influences. That can become clear if we come to an original cosmic way of thinking about the human being.

Now you will recall, on the one hand, the reflections on development which you can find in the outline of my *Occult Science* in which the developmental stream is taken through the Saturn, Sun and Moon development, then followed by Earth development. Human beings have actually gone through all these developmental stages and you will have been able to see from what we have said in these days that human beings initially contain the hereditary stream, which acts in the model, and the individual stream which comes from previous lives on earth. The things which are at work in heredity go back to earlier times but have ahrimanically been left behind, have withered. So that is what lies in heredity. That is basically what today's official medicine works with alone and nowhere does it take account of the other side which is developed in the second phase of life between the change of teeth and puberty—the stage in human life which even statistically can be interpreted as the most healthy one because that is when human beings are least able to fall ill. The ability to fall ill is deactivated.

It is tempting to say that today's medicine has no inclination whatsoever to concern itself with health but likes to rummage around in illness. That is to put it in extreme terms but it is true. But to combine oneself with health it is necessary that we truly bring our understanding of the whole cosmos in the human being to the stage of also seeing the cosmos in the human being. For that we need the details which can truly facilitate such a perception of the cosmic development in the human being. After all, human beings still contain the old Saturn development, the old Sun development and the old Moon development. And only when we have understood these three developments preceding Earth development, only then can we understand what we are looking at in the earthly human being. We have so many scientific disciplines today—but we do not have a real Saturn science, a real sun science, a real moon science because in the general life of nature we can no longer recall what was contained in the instinctive original wisdom. So we can no longer come close to what lived in Hippocrates in the strongest way because it has become an empty phrase. That has to be brought back to life. So you will have an important saying sounding across from ancient times but you will not generally pay attention to this ancient saying and least of all pay attention to the wonderful guidance it can give to medicine. It is as follows.

The divine cosmic powers have ordered life by measurement, number and weight. You can find that as a Bible saying. But who today pays attention to such words other than as a general phrase, as if there had once been an ancient cosmic builder who arranged things by measurement, number and weight. But for the physician it is a matter of really finding measurement, number and weight in the human being. Let us look at the nature of Saturn. You see, human beings have the Saturn development within them but we will not of course find this Saturn development in human beings as they actually exist today because they combine all the developmental stages synthetically; they are combined so that the individual ones disappear in the combination, the harmony. But illness calls forth the one or other phenomenon in its particular form. And now the following has to occur, that what I have set out in *Occult Science* is truly grasped, not with reason alone, but is grasped in the way as it is described there: that one feels in everything how during Saturn development a cosmic warmth worked throughout. If we study Saturn development, we have to refer back to the warmth element, we have look towards the warmth element. Saturn acts in human beings and what has been described about Saturn development acts in human beings but it does not come to appearance in human beings on earth if they contain all these things in harmony within one another. But it acts when a person is ill. Then these things separate which are otherwise harmoniously integrated, then the Saturn element acts on its own in fever. We will only get a science of fever if we make it cosmic, if we are willing to go into the way that Saturn acts in human beings. So we really have to understand how the cosmic influences are at work in the phenomenon of fever through the Saturn forces which we have spiritually found soaked into the earth. If we find the Saturn forces everywhere on the earth's surface, distributed most strongly in the lead forces and otherwise everywhere else, we will obtain an inner insight into fever; and we must see therein those things in accordance with which the divine spiritual cosmic order organizes the world through measurement. The measurement of fever expresses the measurement which lives in the cosmic order when warmth streams into the cosmic order, the measurement which merges and harmonizes with the other aspects. But we have to see measurement above all in the phenomena of fever. Hence we have to let the following strongly work on us: [See Plate 14]

Feel in fever's *measurement*
Saturn's spiritual gift

It is actually the human spirit which appears in fever which is otherwise always submerged in the other elements. The human spirit asserts itself in fever as it becomes one-sided. The oldest component of human nature comes to appearance in fever at the surface of existence.

Now you see, Saturn development is followed by sun development. There the pure warmth element is densified into air on the one hand and diluted into light on the other. Light and air interact, they belong together. We take in the rhythm of air in breathing, light we take in. And light in an occult sense is not just what acts in the eye but light is a general expression for what acts through the sun. It is merely that the eye is the best representative for what acts through the sun. In the Middle Ages, the things which act through light were described as spiritual tincture. Now when we come to sun development we also have sun development in human beings today and we experience it directly as something which does not act on earth, but which is the after-effect of the action of the old Sun, when we place our fingers on a person's pulse and feel it in the right way. The pulse rate expresses the old Sun development in us. And so we have as a second thing:

> Feel in the pulse beat's *number*
> The *sun's* soul power

It is not a matter of indifference, dear friends, whether or not we do the right thing in this regard. We can take such matters seriously or not. But it makes a tremendous difference if, as you read the thermometer with devotion, you truly reflect on the picture which evolution presents at the time of Saturn—this is something that just has to be learned through inner practice: since everything is subject to its streaming warmth, the whole world will appear to you as a spiritual gift in which love streams into each individual thing through that warmth. And if you recognize in this mood of religious devotion how love streams into the world with the assistance of warmth through the nature of Saturn; if you recognize in such thankful devotion to warming, loving cosmic creation; if you recognize in the moment when you check the temperature from out of this mood what is at work, then you will receive an intuition about what you should do.

Equally we should not check someone's pulse in the workman, butcher-like way that it is often done; but with the pulse we should be able to immerse ourselves in what comes from the sun as cosmic rhythm. When feeling a pulse we should be able to feel the immersion of the human being in the brightness which spreads air and light and illuminates the world. Then it is again the case that the whole human being is engaged in the will to heal. The will to heal cannot be brought about through an inner commandment but it can only be achieved if the soul's attitude is one of devotion in the world.

And if you then proceed to check the other symptoms, you will look at the extent to which the things which are at work in human beings do not take human form but their own form. Take the different types of diabetes, for example. What are they based on? On the fact that sugar has not been penetrated fully by human nature, as happens in the harmonized human being, so that the latter does not act through his or her own power; the human being becomes too weak to penetrate sugar fully right down into the very atoms. The human I-organization follows the sugar forces, the extra-human forces. Look at all the forces at work in the human being in diabetes mellitus, which appear in the residues of urine, which are deposited in the body in migraine and other conditions. If you look at all the things which appear in the body as substances which follow their own laws and not the laws of the human being you can pose two questions.

First, how is it possible at all that there can be a tendency in human nature to allow substances to work independently within the human being? If that were not the case, Moon evolution could never have intervened. It intervenes precisely when the substances in human beings want to follow their own path. Then the moon forces take hold of the forces of these substances and, in their capacity as moon forces, bring about the human form. Everything that appears in human beings as form is penetrated by the moon forces. Just as Saturn warms us through and the sun penetrates us with rhythm, the moon gives form to human beings. So you see, that is what the whole human being is like. Remember what I have always emphasized. Our brain does not have its own weight. If we take it out it weighs about 1500 grams but in the body it only weighs about 20 grams because according to the Archimedes principle every body loses as much in weight as the weight of the water it displaces. Now, because it floats in the cerebrospinal fluid, the brain displaces a part of the fluid, giving it buoyancy, so that the downward pressure is only about 20 grams of weight. That is how it is with everything. The forces have to be there in the cosmos to take the weight off human beings to the degree necessary for the substances they have within themselves. Weight has to be regulated and the third element lies in the weight of our own substances and their regulation through the cosmos. So, whether you are investigating whether a substance at work in the metabolism occurs under its own weight or whether it forms part of the weight of the cosmos, you are investigating the order of the divine-spiritual world by weight, which gives you the third element:

> Feel in substance's *weight*
> The moon's *forming power*:

That is the mood which should fill us once again. We should be able to feel when we talk about rheumatism, gout, obstipation, about diabetes, about migraine, about all the conditions which are somehow connected with such deposits which make the separate weights of the substances appear—we should experience how something occurs in our feeling which can be expressed in the words: earthly weight has taken hold of human beings. A lot is contained in such words. Imbue your examinations with such feelings. Just think of the abstract, butcher-like way these examinations are carried out today, with what little thought! Then you will obtain what is missing today, what has been killed off today in Arabism and Islam despite all the ancient wisdom, ancient virtues, ancient skills which have been so wonderfully conserved—killed off because the trinity of moon, sun and Saturn appeared hidden, masked as Father, Son and Holy Spirit, and because this trinity disappeared and because Arabism and Islam simply rejected all those things with the words—I am referring to the words which came before, which Muhammad[48] did not speak but which the angel spoke who inspired him, who was not exactly an admirable angel despite being very wise: Trinity? What Trinity? There is only *one* god whom Muhammad should proclaim. That is what we are referred to, to the disappearance of all differentiation in the world. In that way the things which should actually be known about have been obscured and our medicine has become an Arabic and Islamic one. European humanity had become too weak to find the right thing. We have to know about these things today otherwise humanity on earth will perish, so that you must tell yourselves:

> Feel in fever's *measurement*
> *Saturn's* spiritual gift
> Feel in the pulse beat's *number*
> The *sun's* soul power
> Feel in substance's *weight*
> The moon's *forming power*:
> Then you will also see in your will to heal
> What requires healing in *earthly* human beings.

You see, if we look at the world in this way we have to grasp these things truly with our mind. Then we will develop a sense that there is a tendency in the course of a person's life on earth for the individuality which comes across from previous earth lives to take hold of what exists like a model from the hereditary stream. I have already mentioned the struggle between what is formed in accordance with the model as the second human body, on the one hand, and the first model-like human body, on the other. If we know that we have a human being before us who is working his or her way to the surface then we know that something is at work on this human being which has come from earlier incarnations. And it is truly the case that the person who penetrates these things with his or her heart and soul has the best opportunity to perceive in the sick person what has come across from earlier incarnations, or at least to have an inkling of it.

Because what is it that underlies what comes to expression in illness? In healthy people it is like this. We have the head organization which in its basic form is even externally separated from the remaining organization. The head is a bony casing in which the brain is enclosed. The continuation of the head is also enclosed in bones. It exists by itself and then the rest of what belongs to the human being is connected to it. But there is also something in the finer organization of the human being which separates these two sections from one another. You see, this cannot be shown so easily through outer anatomy and outer physiology, but an enormous amount can be observed in what exists, for example, in the transformation of food substances so that these nutritional substances as they are in their inner structure do not enter the head organization, or indeed the nervous organization. There is a sharply delineated barrier which cannot be crossed. Which must not be crossed by whom? Well, you see, the power from previous lives on earth which has been preserved through the period between death and a new birth works most strongly in the head organization from the start of the human being's development on earth. What is at work as the child's power of individuality comes from the head. But it is not allowed down into the remaining physical organization unscreened. There must be a screen, an intermediate layer. It is not externally visible but it is there in the organization. Nothing goes down unscreened. The lung as an organ or the liver as an organ must not be directly taken hold of by what has come across as forces from earlier incarnations; they cannot cope with it. And something quite terrible happens in human beings when the power from earlier lives on earth comes into contact with, say, the liver unscreened. In the time between death and a new birth, the human individuality transforms the forces which lie in the lungs and liver, in the limb and metabolic system, partly also in the rhythmical system, into head organization. Then the limb and metabolic organization must be attached again from the outside. The human individuality, which is eternal, may only enter it again once the human being has passed through the portal of death when the physical and material part falls away and only the forces of lung and liver have passed through the portal of death. Thus harm arises in human beings during their life on earth if the individuality enters certain organs which it should not.

That is why, on the basis of inner devotion, we say with regard to certain medical conditions: oh, here the individuality from the previous life on earth is acting on the organ which now should only be influenced by this earth life because there is no separation. That is why you see the action of the individuality from a previous earth life in sick people. This individuality—which should exist only in the moral sphere, the sphere of destiny, which should stop at what human beings do and learn and which should not touch the organization in the mainly earthly part of the human being—works partly in the metabolic and limb system, partly in the rhythmical system, partly in the nervous and sensory system because the barrier has become damaged. You see, a way of approaching human beings arises when we know that the individuality of the human being is at work in the diseased lung. When I look at someone with pulmonary consumption, I feel a very concrete empathy because our time is so materialistic and distracts the human being in the external world from how his or her karma should be lived out through destiny, pushes him or her morally back into the physical body because of our whole unspiritual life. Instead of passing over into the moral sphere, the individuality rejects our time. It becomes organic, takes hold of the organs, takes hold above all of the lung which is the inward facing aspect of the metabolic and limb system, which in turn faces outwards. The individuality intervening from earlier incarnations takes hold directly of the body. These things are not of such importance because we can theorize about them but because we can put ourselves in that position with our whole frame of mind and then the will to heal arises which is in turn connected in the right way with a person's need for healing. In our present materialistic culture there is actually an exceptionally sharp division between the healing person and the person seeking healing. They cannot connect because more is needed to create a connection, because we have to have a feeling for what lives in human beings as the eternal part. And on the basis of such a feeling the right relationship develops between the healer and the person seeking healing and then we can develop a sense of how we must truly individualize; because each person has his or her own karma. We must individualize in the healing process.

These are the things, you see, which we should let act on our mind. These things become esoteric when we let them act on our mind and something like the Gospel of Luke contains all of the mood we require to progress in this feeling. That is why it is the case that these things have come about objectively. Four faculties have come about, a Luke faculty, a Matthew faculty, a Mark faculty and a John faculty, but we see nothing of that today because Arabism lives particularly in medicine. The permeation with Christianity will take place when we grasp things in such a way that we return to the cosmic. Then you also have to be conscious of your cosmic position as physicians. You will have seen from all this the extent to which the regulating forces of the moon affect the human form. If the moon's regulating forces in the human form are too irregular in their action, then we have to direct our mind to that, then we have to be clear that we heal by removing the bit of irregularity which lives in the form; and that happens when we treat the sick person in such a way that cosmic awareness is also involved. But then, you see, something else must become clear. We have to gain a perspective. You must look at something from the outside. After all, you cannot look at the eye from the outside. Those things which allow us to look at everything from the outside, which are at work there, are the things which on the other hand give us clear concepts about everything and do not immediately involve abstraction in these clear concepts but let our heart think along. We must not become confused in our concepts but neither must we exclude the heart from our abstract thinking. We must be human beings by being whole human beings, by the heart always thinking along. Hence we must endeavour not just to think our way into the world, to think our way abstractly into it, which basically all thinking does today. We must be clear that we have to immerse ourselves with our thinking, that the heart has to be involved in everything. We must also know what warmly coils itself around the thoughts; we have to learn to handle Mercury's staff again and we cannot do it in any other way [See Plate 15] than to move from the moon to Mercury. That is what I meant with regard to general culture in the lectures which also dealt with Raphael[49] because Raphael is indeed the Christian Mercury.

If you imbue yourself with such an awareness you will develop the right feelings for the things which you have to work for if you want to enter medicine as young people today. Everywhere in the world the opposite of what should be happening in substance is welling up, and particularly with regard to medicine something terrible has developed in recent times. That is—please forgive me for descending to something mundane, but it shows how the opposite acts—that is the medical health insurance system. It has cut out the physician primarily. In Germany there is an expression which testifies to the exclusion of the human element in the physician, which testifies to the view that abstraction is at work here and not the human being. In reality it is the physician who heals and not medical science. But people think that medical science is something that floats about independently of the person. The human being is left out of consideration—it is a downright slap in the face for karma. Karma works in such a way that it does not blindly link up one person with another but in fact a karmic element comes to expression in the free choice of physician, where that is possible. But the purely ahrimanic set-up of health insurance panel doctors leaves karma completely out of the picture and human beings are exposed to the ahrimanic powers which do nothing but fight karma. When we meet again I will tell you how the ahrimanic powers are intent on killing human karma so that they can achieve their goal. But that is inherent in the health insurance system and the institution of not being free to choose one's physician; and it merely indicates, does it not, what comes to expression in language in the choice of the term 'health care industry'. I believe it is even used in the law on health insurance companies. That is symptomatic of the whole outlook which is inherent in the health insurance system and the view of the medical system as a 'health care industry'. In a sign of the times it is a symptom of the emergence of the cultural disease which also appears in many other guises today and which attests to the way in which physicians in particular must help to heal these cultural diseases. But if a physician is put in a position in which he or she is himself or herself subjected to this cultural disease in the severest way, the physician is completely paralysed. And just think that this is the most terrible fact represented in the institution of the health insurance funds. They also have their good sides, of course, in the way that the things which emerge in the world and aim to tempt and mislead people appear to be nice and shiny and not something that we necessarily dislike. The devil always appears in the guise of an angel. Anyone who sees the devil in the shape of the devil in their vision can be sure that it is not the devil because the latter appears in the shape of an angel. If physicians are subject to the most severe impulse of a cultural disease, then our culture is basically on the way to being sick. That is why it is necessary for you to take note of your karma and where it places you in order to work not just in the medical field but also on the sick nature of the social organism.

So please formulate your questions with that in mind. We will meet once more tomorrow. I have also heard that you have a certain desire for an explanation as to how you can integrate into the general youth movement. We will be able to supplement a number of the things which I spoke about in particular today. But I did want to say what I said today because I thought that it might be necessary for you to know and digest.

> Feel in fever's *measurement*
> *Saturn's* spiritual gift
> Feel in the pulse beat's *number*
> The *sun's* soul power
> Feel in substance's *weight*
> The moon's *forming power*:
> Then you will also see in your will to heal
> What requires healing in *earthly* human beings.

MY dear friends,
Today I would still like to tell you a number of things following on from
the observations we have made and then speak a little about the general
subject to which your individual questions relate. I now want to say
something which it was better to leave until we had obtained the kind of
knowledge we have discussed in the last few days. Specifically, it is
necessary to avoid putting general truths at the beginning of one's
observations and to move on to general truths only once one has gained
some experience because only in that way does the general acquire its
true and real coloration. So now let us consider that the four components of human nature, the physical body, etheric body, astral body
and I, each have their own special structure. The physical and etheric
bodies have a structure in space and time, the astral body and I a purely
spiritual structure. We have to imagine a purely spiritual structure by
telling ourselves: a spiritual structure has no space or time. Space and
time have gone. But I can create an image for myself of the spiritual
structure and imagine it that way. That takes place in the imaginative
consciousness. But you now have to remember that we are dealing with
a physical and etheric structure on the one hand, which is completely
separated from the spiritual and soul structure in the sleeping human
being, and on the other hand with a certain spiritual and soul structure.

You see, when we look at the sleeping human being, we have a
pronounced physical and etheric structure in such sleeping human
beings who have sent their I and astral body away. And we have, in

turn, the soul and spiritual structure separately from the physical and etheric body. They are very different from one another. The physical and etheric structure is differentiated into the individual organs as an organism which has, we might say, brought forth the individual organs as if from the centre of life. The astral and I structure are much more driven from the outside to the inside, that is, arise more through invagination; so the important thing here is that space and time are left out through invagination. The key thing is that the two are fundamentally different from one another, the physical and etheric and the spiritual and soul structure. Now the spiritual and soul entity, the astral and I-organization, is—if we use an expression which is not quite correct but illustrates the matter—engaged in the physical and etheric organization in human beings when they are in the physical world in a waking state. They penetrate one another to a certain degree. So in every physical organ which is warmed through and filled with light by its etheric body, and also filled with life in that the cosmos works through the etheric body, in each physical organ we do have the intervention of the I-organization and astral organization in the human being when awake. Now simply consider the following. The I-organization and astral organization force their own structure on a given organ or organ system. In other words, something that should have a physical and etheric structure receives a spiritual structure, becomes an image of the astral and I-organization. That is basically the universal cause of physical illness. Speaking in universal terms, the cause of physical illness is this, that a person's body becomes too spiritual in a given location or as a whole. That is why the proper, dedicated observation of the sick human being is so immensely enlightening—as was observed particularly strongly in ancient times—for understanding the spiritual human being. Just remember, in ancient times when people felt quite differently about human nature from the way they do now—I therefore do not say the following to resurrect the desire in some way that we should return to such methods today—but in ancient times when people had more robust views about the human being this was also expressed through phenomena such as these. If it was deemed necessary for the salvation of people with heretical views, they were burnt. They were burnt, allegedly at least for their salvation, these heretics, so that they would be liberated from what would otherwise deliver them into terrible torments after their death. That was a kind of vision in earlier times which then turned into brutality. People had more robust views about the human being and as a result it could happen that a person whom we would consider to be healthy was given Melissa in a specific preparation. If they were given Melissa in a particular way, their consciousness was pervaded with a touch of dreaminess. They became more dreamy than they were otherwise before being given Melissa, but as a result subtle imaginations lodged in their consciousness. If they were treated with Hyoscyamus, for example, in a certain way, then they would develop a strong tendency for Inspiration. The following was found, for example, through such investigations. It was found that if the solar plexus was stimulated with Hyoscyamus the solar plexus was pervaded with spirit. It was found that then the astral body and I-organization intervened strongly in the solar plexus. Or it was noticed that the whole blood supply to the cerebrum increased by a small degree—which had a very important effect however—if the person was given Melissa juice—because the I-organization intervenes strongly through the cerebral cortex. And so the whole human being was examined as to the way that he or she could become spiritual and how the individual organs showed how they could become more spiritual. It is a preconception that we think with the head. That is not true at all. We think with the legs and the arms; and the head watches what happens in the arms and the legs and assimilates it in the images of the thoughts. It would never—I already told you about that in the Christmas course—get to know the law of the angle without walking. It would never become familiar with the mechanical laws of equilibrium if it did not learn about them through its own centre of gravity which it carries about in the subconscious. As soon as we get down to the astral body, which processes all these things in the subconscious, human beings appear incredibly wise, even if they sometimes are quite foolish in the physical world; because all the things which develop as geometry through walking, through a feeling of self, for example, because all these things are—if I may be so paradoxical—known in the sub-conscious and are then looked at by the brain. Now you see, if the spiritual and soul organization intervenes too strongly in the physical and etheric organization, physical illness arises. And in the past the spirit was simply investigated through the physical organs because all the things which we can refer to as being a gift from above are spiritual, are soul and spirit. But now we have to make a distinction with regard to what human beings received as a gift from above by purely spiritual means. That continued to be called a gift. But let us take an example, Belladonna.

It is usually the physical and etheric which are at work in plants, but in Belladonna cosmic astrality is coming in most powerfully from outside. And in all the instances in which the spiritual acts on plants or animals—either the astral or what corresponds to the I-organization in the cosmos—poisons are created in contrast to spiritual gifts. But they are certainly the correlate of the spiritual because they are those things in the plants and animals which go beyond the plantlike and are cosmic and astral. When we introduce the astral through Hyoscyamus, we are simply introducing what lives in the warmth cover of the earth, with which the atmosphere ends, into the human solar plexus and also into the human diaphragm. But when we take Melissa, which is not an actual poison, then we get this slight spiritual effect which only comes to expression in a dazed feeling. We might say that in Melissa the poison is in a nascent state. That leads you to the rule: physical illness is when the physical organism or its parts become too spiritualized. Now something else can also happen. It can happen that while human beings are awake, the spiritual and soul structure of their astral body or I-organization enter a physical organ too strongly. But now they do not impose their spiritual and soul structure on the physical organism through their strength but, on the contrary, have the physical structure imposed on them by the physical organism; so that when human beings are asleep the astral body and I become copies of the physical and etheric body so that human beings take the physical structure into their astral body and I. You see, these two ways in which irregularities can occur in human beings are substantially different from one another, also in terms of what we observe. In an ill person the diseased organ becomes remarkably spiritualized. It becomes brighter. It is visible as if the spiritual had caught hold of it from the outside in, from the surface. For the occult gaze, an ill person appears transparent, I might say, long before there are any clear signs in the colour of the skin and suchlike, and this transparency is penetrated by the soul and spiritual entity. In people in which the other is the case, that the soul and spiritual organization takes on the structure of the physical and etheric, it can be noticed by way of the soul and spiritual entity in the way that such people sleep: in that situation they become a wraith, a light, breezy wraith of their physical body. They continue to resemble their physical body. They really do become a spectre of their physical body. And the crude experiments conducted by spiritists in so-called manifestations are all based on this—what I say does happen in some hidden way—that the soul and spiritual entity is weakened in a medium. That is also obvious. Then in the dark room—it is also the case otherwise—the weakened astral body and the weakened I can take on the forms of the organs to the point where they become visible in the dark room so that although the manifestations are true they are also nefarious. Now all so-called mental illnesses are based on the spiritual and soul entity, the astral body and I-organization, taking on the physical and etheric structure. That is the basis for all so-called mental illness so that you can say: physical illness is based on the spiritualization of the physical organism or its parts; mental illness is based on the astral or I-organization or their parts taking physical or etheric form. That is a general truth which provides exceptional guidance for human understanding.

That is something which relates, in turn, to questions which some have asked with regard to the relationship between medicine and education. For we have all the degrees between these two extremes before us in the child's organism. In the one child, the astral and I-organization may have the greater tendency to spiritualize the physical body and etheric body, in another child they may have the greater tendency to have their form specified by the physical and etheric; and there are all possible intermediate stages in between. This basic law is in turn reflected in the temperaments. If it is the case that the astral body and the I-organization have the very strong, intense tendency—not yet to the point of insanity, so that a person can still manage—but the intense tendency to take on forms from the physical or etheric body, then we are dealing with a melancholic temperament. In the instant in which the astral body and the I-organization have the tendency to impress their own structure strongly on the physical or etheric body, we are dealing with the choleric temperament. And the phlegmatic and sanguine temperaments lie in between. In the phlegmatic temperament it is the case that the astral body and the I-organization do not have such an intense tendency, but to a certain extent have the tendency to assume the structure of the physical and, particularly, the etheric body. In the sanguine temperament it is the case that the vitality which lies in the etheric body is strongly influenced by the astral body. That is how it is also expressed in the temperaments. And we can see how what in radical cases can provide guidance for physicians—recognizing how in the waking person the soul and spiritual entity is engaged with the physical and etheric—is also the rule for the educator in its latent states so that actually education and medicine are things which continue one into the other. The thing is, my dear friends, to seek as much as possible to reach Imagination in looking at the human being. Now I would still like to give you some points of reference particularly with that in mind.

You can picture for yourself, at least that knowledge is available to you, you can picture for yourself the form of the human being in the embryonic state. Today people have obtained, as far as that is possible, a view of the embryonic state in the initial stages and how it develops later on, and on that basis you can obtain a coherent picture of the human being in the embryonic state. You can further obtain a coherent picture of the human being during the childhood stage. You must try to visualize the first and the second picture as intensely as possible so that you really scan it with your thinking, so that it really appears to you as if you were scanning the embryo with your thinking, inwardly tracing its forms. Then you enlarge the embryo to this size [hand movement], simply in your thinking to the size which the child has which you can look at, observe with equal intensity. And then you insert your mental image, the picture of the embryo into the picture of the child by inwardly metamorphosing it. You will have some difficulties in your inner experience if you do it properly. You will have to tell yourself: 'If I take the head of the embryo and enlarge it to the childhood stage, then it will become very large. I then have to compress it. I also have to inwardly crystallize and coagulate what is still watery fluid in the embryo, is strongly a part of the fluid human being, in order for that to become the brain of the embryo.' And then you will take the embryonic state of the limbs, will have to stretch and form them, will have to undertake an inward sculptural activity and insert the unshaped limbs of the embryo into the limbs of the child. It is an exceptionally interesting inner occupation to insert the embryo into childhood age in your inner perception.

Then you can go further. Then you can take the child and the adult and do the same experiment with them. That becomes more difficult. The differences between the embryo and the child are very great; you will need to develop great inner activity if you do that. But if you now compare childhood with the adult state in the mature human being, then the differences are not so great. It becomes somewhat difficult to fit the one with the other. But if you manage to proceed in this way, then the imagination of the human etheric body truly is born in you; the imagination of the human etheric body is born relatively quickly.

Take note:

> Push the early years

—embryonic period—

> Into childhood
> And childhood
> Into adolescence:
> You will see condensed
> Human etheric existence
> Behind bodily nature

—the physical body in its structure.

There you have a guiding rule which you can use just as well as the others which I spoke about yesterday and in the first session. You just have to understand clearly with all of them that the acquisition of the imaginative consciousness requires effort. You cannot obtain it by magic but have to acquire it through intensive work.

Now you can go even further. You can attempt to imagine an ancient person, an ancient sclerotic person. Ancient people are sclerotic to a certain degree. And if you develop the feeling that you are also scanning this ancient person, you will get the impression in that spiritual scan penetrating the sclerosis that the ancient person is actually hollow. So you do not get the impression that a sclerotic ancient person is denser, harder when you scan him or her but, on the contrary, that he or she is not harder at all but actually sucks inwards. As you scan that person spiritually you get the same feeling as when you physically rub a wet finger over meerschaum [hydrated magnesium silicate or sepiolite]. You know of course that when you rub a wet finger over clay or sepiolite you get that feeling of suction. This feeling of suction is what you get with regard to the ancient sclerotic person. You have to develop this sense of scanning, this experiential feeling with regard to your perception. That is not only the case when looking with the eye but with every sense, including the life sense. So you now have the density of age, which sucks in, when you understand this. Now you push—just as you pushed forwards in the first case from the embryonic stage into childhood and then into the mature human being—so you now push backwards. Imagine the mature human being, who does not yet suck in but who stands strongly in the world, and push what you have scanned in the spirit into that human being. When you push the embryonic structure into the childhood structure, you undertake a spatial metamorphosis; now, when it appears to you as if the ancient person is a hollowed out being which is continuously sucking inwards, you have to act as if that being were filled with strength when it is pushed backwards into the mature period of life. We become the mature person by pushing it back. Whereas previously, when we are looked at bristling with strength, we perceive something of a slight paralysis, the ancient person when pushed backwards like this grows strong in his or her bones again and in the whole structure of his or her solid organism. This inner way of pushing one thing into another has to be observed to a greater extent and then the mature age also has to be pushed back into youth. That is actually easy again. Imagine a person who already has a wrinkled face and let him fuse with a young, chubby person; that will create balance. If we can manage that, then we gain the impression as if waves were moving through the etheric body and it started to sound. That is how we get an impression of the astral in the human being.

So you have a rule which guides you to rise to Inspiration: [See Plate 16]

> Push the density of age
> Into the period of human maturity
> And the age of maturity
> Into the life of youth.
> You will hear resound in cosmic sound
> Human soul activity

—that is the astral body—

Out of etheric life.

You can see from what I have said that the instructions for meditation are not given as orders but are based on insight. The person guided to meditation in the right way is not treated in the authoritarian way that used to be the case in the ancient East where the education and development both of children and older people was based on quite different foundations from ours. So anyone who is recommended meditations by us is given them in such a way that they understand what they do with themselves. You see, in the East children were instructed by their dada. That meant that the children were brought up and educated through the way that the person concerned lived. They did not learn more than they could copy from the dada. Adults had their guru if they wanted to progress further. In that situation they were dependent on their guru whose only rule was: this is how it is—do it. That is the difference. What we have in our Western civilization is that an appeal is everywhere made to the freedom of the individual, that people know what they are doing. And we can understand how inspired understanding comes about when we have understood with our sound common sense how physical illness and mental illness work and when we compare what I have told you today. Because all these things can be understood with sound common sense. If we go further in order to understand what to do in inner meditation, then we have come to the limits of what we can attain with sound common sense. Sound common sense can attain everything that comes from anthroposophy. At the point where those things start which can no longer be attained with sound common sense, then it has worked properly to its limits and it is like standing at a lake. That is a similar kind of limit; one can continue to look from the edge of the lake. Sound common sense does, truly, takes us to all these things. You must not fall prey to the slur that you are spreading a mystical, obscure world view, but one that can be attained with sound common sense. When I said that once in Berlin I was criticized in an article about the lecture which said: sound common sense cannot understand anything of the spiritual world; and anyone who understands anything about the spiritual world is sick, is not healthy. That was the argument used against me.

Now I still want to say something about the fact that you are in a very special position as young people because you are required through your medical studies to look deeply into the whole nature and essence of the human being. You see, we have to take very seriously that the Kali Yuga has come to an end, that we have entered an age of light, even if humanity still lives in darkness because the old continues through inertia. Something bright is shining in from the spiritual cosmos and as human beings we are entering an age of light and people only have to open themselves to receiving the intentions of the age of light. Now young people are indeed predestined to grow into the age of light; and if these young people develop a certain self-awareness with the requisite seriousness as to why they are in the position of having been born precisely at the start of the age of light, then these young people will have the opportunity in various degrees to fit in with what is required by the developmental impulse of humanity. And that requires today that we look to the human being in all respects if we want to explain the world, just as previously people looked to nature to assemble the human being out of the individual forces and processes of nature. We will gradually have to reach the stage of understanding the human being, and comprehending the individual processes in nature as specializations, one-sided manifestations of what happens in the human being. If we manage that, a certain intimate relationship will take hold in all of human feeling and mind activity which has been sought, but sought in a certain tumultuous way. Just think how young people started to idolize nature in a certain way when the youth movement of the age of light came along. It was abstract; however great the vitality with which it was felt, it was abstract. In contrast, the spiritual path of development of young people today must lead to deep feelings regarding their connection as human beings with the world, deep feelings, and what they assimilate spiritually must no longer be science for the intellect. That leaves us cold; people have always been left cold by that. Science must develop in such a way that something really does occur in the sense that with every stage we achieve in science we also change as human beings in our mind, in our feelings, that we become acquainted with something we have forgotten. After all, we did become acquainted with nature, for example, before we came down into the physical world. But it looked different then. Today what young people went through in their previous existence is killed off when we refer them to crude, robust external perception. Once it occurs to people to treat external sensory perception as if an old acquaintance turned up in sensory perception whom we know from pre-earthly life, then feeling will enter knowledge, feeling will enter cognition in all instances. And this must truly be like a bloodstream, like a spiritual bloodstream which flows through all of scientific life, through human education and teaching as such. This intimate relationship with what is real—that is what we have to obtain in science.

In this respect the modern age was truly overloaded with concepts. You see, I tried to show at a relatively early stage how human beings, when they see the external world of the senses, actually only have half of reality; how they can only obtain the whole of reality when they combine what arises in them and external sensory reality. And I had to start with that because the time was quite different then from today. Things are still in preparation. I had to set it out epistemologically. But if you read my work *Truth and Knowledge*[50] you will work towards letting the spiritual arise in the human mind, a spiritual which springs up from the inside. That is the first step towards such a deepening of science, particularly towards accepting cosmic reality in heart and mind. Now that is something which is particularly possible for physicians, that they learn about such intimate experience of reality; and that is why physicians—just because they are physicians—will be the people capable of turning the abstractness of the rest of the youth movement, those who are not destined to be physicians, into a more concrete form with inwardness of heart and mind. After all, it is possible as young people who have medicine within them to deepen the medical, as we are doing here, with other people who, for example, only have jurisprudence within them and are poor fellows because they only have jurisprudence; with jurists it is quite impossible. Something of the spirit was still present in medicine until the early eighteenth century; in jurisprudence the spiritual ceased as long ago as deep in the Middle Ages, and people no longer even have the slightest inkling of spirit but only of statutory notices. It is quite possible for physicians, who are the first to enter concrete life, to have an exceptionally fruitful effect on other young people.

That is why it would be a good thing if the individual groups which have emerged in the anthroposophical youth movement were to be supported by the physicians in particular. Of course we have to take account of the existing karmic conditions. But we have the very hopeful Tuebingen group, which is working with education, and which will be able to gain a great deal, for example, if it has a physician in it who can clarify things with regard to the medical side. Here we now have Dr Bockholt[51] leading the youth movement, even if only on an interim basis, and it will be a very good thing if the youth movement is fertilized by what develops inwardly in physicians. And so we can do extra-ordinarily much in individual instances. But on the other hand it would also be good if you occasionally, when the possibility arises, were to concern yourself as much as possible with the educational work in the anthroposophical movement. If there is a serious approach, there is no obstacle to prevent you from concerning yourself with that, but in a serious way. What is presented in the seminars of the Waldorf school cannot be given to everyone. But when someone demonstrates that they are concerned seriously with the subject, there can be no obstacle to becoming familiar with the seminar courses of the Waldorf school when these things are also truly viewed from the medical side; and also inwardly penetrated with the thought of the close relationship between healing and education in antiquity.

Just consider that today we have completely abandoned the view of the human being as an entity who enters earth life afflicted with sin because the modern view no longer has any idea of what sin means. What has been consolidated into the concept of sin? What I demon-

strated to you in these days as the law of heredity is based on sin, on
original sin. And individual sin is also something that human beings
have to overcome in the second half of their lives. They must properly
overcome the sinful model which originates from heredity—we can also
say from the sick model in accordance with the old concepts. But if
human beings kept as their body what is at work in the model up to the
change of teeth, if they bore that for the whole of their life, they would
be a person at nine years of age who—well, whose skin would be
covered in weeping eczema if the organization continued like that; they
would get holes in their whole body, would look like a leper, the flesh
would fall off their bones if they were able to bear it at all. Human
beings are born sick into the world and education means recognizing
and guiding what works in accordance with the model, means the same
as subtle healing. You should live in the youth movement with the
awareness that when you describe education you consider yourselves as
therapists. You specify the medicines which of course remain in the
spiritual but can have a strong physical effect depending on how much
the child passes into the pathological. That is what you basically have in
education, but only at a different level, on a different plane—also a
healing art. And, on the other hand, if the patient does not want to help
in any way through what he can be given as guidance for his own
subjective awareness of the illness, for pessimism or optimism regarding
his view of life, if it is impossible to work educationally, it is incredibly
difficult to support him in a way that brings healing. If the patient—I
do not want to say that he should have a blind belief in the medicine,
that would be an exaggeration—but if the patient is brought to the
point simply through the individuality of the physician that he
experiences how the physician is permeated with the will to heal, there is
a reflex in the patient which is then permeated by the will to be healthy.
This powerful coming together of the will to heal and the will to be
healthy plays a tremendously great role in treatment so that we can
indeed say: it contains an image of education and education contains an
image of healing. A great deal depends today on people finding one
another in the world in the right state of mind. So if young people in
medicine come together with the other young people in the right
consciousness, then you will see that the young people in medicine can

have an exceptionally fruitful effect on the others. But sharpening your awareness towards both sides in this way is a particular necessity.

You see, these are the things I would like to place in your soul and your heart, now that you have been here once again in such a satisfactory way. I hope it has contributed again to strengthening and making closer the bonds between your souls and the Goetheanum and that you feel that particularly in such a concrete field as medicine the Goetheanum finds the people to carry out into the world what can be found here. You will develop a proper awareness of that if you also consider yourself as part of the Goetheanum in your feelings and frequently direct your thoughts to what the Goetheanum wants to achieve for the world and the development of our civilization. And so the bonds of the heart which you can tie with the Goetheanum will be something which can help you in a profound way with the task you have set yourselves specifically as physicians. It is with this feeling in mind that I particularly wanted to hold these more intimate discussions as we have done in these sessions here, and I believe that we will be able to achieve a considerable amount if you continue with this feeling, which has permeated these discussions in particular, out into the world, now that we have had to hold the last session today. And in that way we will stay together in the nicest way. The Goetheanum will be able to see itself as the centre in the best possible way which has set itself a particular task. The Goetheanum will thereby truly be the Goetheanum and you will be true Goetheanists. Then you will simultaneously be the supporting pillars outside in the world which the Goetheanum needs and from this perspective I appeal to your soul to become true and proper Goetheanists. If we do it in that way, everything will turn out well.

> Push the early years
> Into childhood
> And childhood
> Into adolescence:
> You will see condensed
> Human etheric existence
> Behind physical nature

Push the density of age
Into the period of human maturity
And the age of maturity
Into the life of youth.
You will hear resound in cosmic sound
Human soul activity
Out of etheric life.

FIRST NEWSLETTER

following the Christmas course
for those committed to medicine[52]

DEAR Friends,   Goetheanum, 11 March 1924

In compliance with what we promised on the occasion of the Christmas conference about the way the Medical Section at the Goetheanum was to be managed, we send this first newsletter to those who are connected with us in the cultivation of medicine. It is carried by the sentiment which united us at the medical courses at New Year. It would like nothing better than to include with each word something of the feeling for suffering humanity from which alone must come not just the devotion to healing but also its real power.

> In ancient times
> There lived in the soul of initiates
> Powerfully the thought that each person
> Is ill by nature.
> And education was seen
> As being equal to the healing process
> Which gave children, as they matured,
> Also the health
> For full humanity in life.

It is good to contemplate such powerful thoughts—obtained from the perception of ancient instinctual wisdom—in the soul if we want to prepare the soul to grasp the effects of healing in the right kind of inner composure.

Let us not forget that the healing process has to be accompanied by a soul because it has to address not just a body but also a soul. The more young physicians understand such thoughts, the more those things will flow into medical life which the thoughtful physician is longing for when he or she experiences the state of his or her art with its limitations, and which the patient will experience as a blessing when he or she experiences it in the healing process.

Dear friends, those of you who were gathered here in January accepted with an open heart what sought you out on the basis of such sentiments. We will never forget how this was reflected in your eyes, how we encountered it in your warm words. Our thoughts were with you and today they go to you for the first time in response to the questions you have asked.

We will send the following to individual addresses and ask those who receive direct mailings from us to make sure that they are forwarded to the addresses notified by us.

*

Goetheanum, 11 March 1924

Questions and Answers

I.   In response to a question regarding the difficulties which the prospective physician encounters both in the study of conventional medicine and the medical courses in the anthroposophical movement, we can only reply that it will precisely be our endeavour to remove these difficulties in the course of time through the communications in these newsletters. Dr Wegman is prepared to give the meditation, which is described as supplementary in the letter, to those who feel a need for it.[53]

II.   Regarding studies at the Goetheanum.
      Practical studies will, of course, be taken care of as far as possible. But we ask for patience in that respect. We will notify the time from which registration is possible in these newsletters.

III. Regarding the question about certain subjects being set for staff of the Medical Section [of the School] of Spiritual Science, we note that we would be happy to take the work in this direction.

But it will be easier to negotiate such subjects through individual correspondence than insertion in this newsletter. But here, too, we ask for a little patience. We will come ever closer to our goals but we can only progress one step at a time. We would also like to add that in future questions that are asked regarding the treatment of very specific cases will not be answered in the newsletter. We welcome, of course, questions of a general therapeutic nature that are asked with regard to the medical courses which have taken place, as well as questions relating to physiological and anatomical problems, to medical studies and to the humane and moral attitude of the physician.

IV.   For those people who asked us whether they could come here in the near future to take part in the work of the School or who—perhaps after passing their exams—have such a wish, we note that three to five additional lectures are to be given directly after the Easter lectures from 19–22 April; the people concerned can in the first instance take guidance from them with regard to their further work. The subject: the nature of the human being and world orientation in the light of education and healing as well as of the initially most important tasks of humanity in this field.

V.   Setting up family medicine chests with our medicines would undoubtedly be desirable but cannot be done at the moment as the law says that only homoeopathic medicines which they have dispensed themselves can be given by government-appointed town physicians. Once we are in the same position as these homoeopathic physicians (i.e. with regard to recognition under law) we will be able to do the same. In the meantime we have to be content with making these medicines available by way of a pharmacy.

VI.   In response to the question as to whether the patient should be told about the way that the medicines work, we can say that the effect is indeed compromised if the knowledge about that is absorbed in the thoughts. But the harm is least if the thoughts are only intellectual, greater if they are in image form, greatest if the patient is capable of following the whole healing process himself or herself. But that should neither prevent giving any information about the effect which is wanted nor deny a knowing patient treatment. Because what is lost through knowledge can be completely won back if the patient develops reverence for the method of treatment. Any information given must ensure that this happens.

VII.   Question about the type of injection.

The injection should, as a rule, be given subcutaneously; only if the patient fails to react after several attempts should the injection be given intravenously in highly potentized doses. In such a case the effect of the first injection must have passed.

VIII.   The letter refers to two lines of which the one runs in the direction of the spine, the other from the head downwards and marks the hyoid bone, mandibular arch, thyroid cartilage, lateral part of the ribs. And the question is about the meaning of these lines. The latter line corresponds to what in animals is formed by the astral body from the most solid substances. In humans this line is given its orientation through the upright posture in which it forms an oblique angle with the vertical. This is guided by the I-organization in such a way that the earthly I has what might be described as a hypertrophic effect along the vertebrae; the developing I, which then remains after death, orientates the cartilaginous part of the ribs and the sternum hypertrophically. Because in spiritual beings like Lucifer the human element is bypassed, both the spine and the cartilage part of the ribs with the sternum are absent. That is why the person who posed the question noticed the pointed chest and ribs inclined to the side on the sculpture of Lucifer.[54]

IX.   With regard to the question about the cavities of the head and their importance, we can say the following. The physical and etheric part of the head are organized in such a way that in certain places the physical and in other places the etheric pre-dominates, and the cavities appear in the latter places. They are the actual vehicles of the thoughts whereas the places which are physically completely developed are the vehicles of life in the head and suppress the thinking life. If their activity is too strong, fainting or hallucinations or similar things occur.

X.   With regard to the question about a mediumistic predisposition. The mediumistic predisposition of a person is based on the failure of the astral body and I fully to engage with the abdominal and limb tract of the etheric and physical body in the trance state. As a result the limbs and abdomen are engaged in an irregular way in the etheric and astral surroundings as kind of sense organs. Spiritual perceptions arise in this way; but at the same time the moral and conventional impulses which are normally at work in these organs are disabled just as they are also disabled in our ordinary sense organs. The eye sees the colour blue but not calumny and defamation. It is extremely difficult to achieve the physical healing of mediums. It could only be brought about through highly potentized tobacco injections into a part of a sense organ, for example into the inner part of the Eustachian tube or the cornea of the eye, which is of course very dangerous. Psychiatric healing requires without fail that the healer has a stronger will than the medium outside the trance and that he or she can work through suggestion in the waking state.

XI.   With regard to the question as to whether one is intervening in the karma of the mother and the karma of the child when a pregnancy is terminated to save the mother, the following can be said: both karmas are steered along a different path for a short period but soon put themselves back on their appropriate course so that in that respect we can hardly talk about an intervention in their karma. By contrast, there is great intervention in the karma of the person undertaking the operation. And that latter has to ask himself or herself whether he or she is willing in full awareness to take on himself or herself something that will create karmic connections which would not have been there without such an intervention. But questions of this kind cannot be answered in general terms but are dependent on the special circumstances of each case, just like some things are also an intervention in karma on a purely soul level in cultural life and can lead to deep, tragic conflicts in life.

XII. A question concerning cod liver oil.
      Cod liver oil can be avoided if what underlies the corresponding

illness is diagnosed and the medicines we have indicated are used:
such as,

Waldon I: vegetable protein, vegetable fat

Waldon II: vegetable protein, vegetable fat, iron silicate

Waldon III: vegetable protein, vegetable fat, iron silicate and
Calcarea carbonica.

XIII.   When people who have suffered an injury have been in touch
with the soil, Belladonna D30 together with Hyoscyamus D15
will be of benefit even if only a single injection is given.

XIV.   Concerning the case of a 35-year-old diabetic.

For this diabetic the rosemary cure would undoubtedly be the
best. It could be further supported by giving silicic acid in
decimal 10.

XV.   A question about the treatment of tinnitus.

For tinnitus, opium in decimal 6 is to be recommended for
general treatment. Psychologically it is possible to bring about
an improvement in time if the person can muster enough
strength to transform the passive surrender to the ringing sound
into active imagination, as if one were causing the sound oneself.
Tinnitus is based on the weakening of the astral body relative to
the etheric body in the bladder region.

XVI.   Question about a case of encephalitis lethargica with sequelae.

One could try injecting the 38-year-old patient suffering the
sequelae of the encephalitis, who did not respond to the medicines used, with fly agaric D30, ensuring that after the injection
there is a confident, cheerful atmosphere.

sig. *Rudolf Steiner*   sig. *Dr I. Wegman*

ADDENDUM TO THE EASTER COURSE
FOR PHYSICIANS

Evening meeting with young physicians

DORNACH, 24 APRIL 1924

Rudolf Steiner gave the following answer in response to a question about the apprehension of the fluid human being through imaginative perception.

Well now, you will not manage very well if you start with the details and not with the general. It really is necessary that you start with such observations from the universal and, above all, follow up the things meditatively which I have already spoken about. You see, if we look at the general context we have in nature—I am only speaking about the things which must gradually lead to an imaginative conception—we have in nature the form of the drop. It is normally considered in such a way that we think of the drop as being held together from the inside. But that is not necessary. We can also think of the drop as being formed from all sides, from the outside. Then we have in the surface of the drop the oneness of the cosmic dimension.

You also of course have to consider in these things that the imaginative conception must aim for the truth and that current ideas which we bring with us from a general education depart as far as is possible from the truth. People imagine today that there is infinite space with the stars scattered inside it. Well, starting with such a conception means taking nothing into account in the most brutal way other than merely what has been thought up. Just take the report in all the papers recently, which should be taken more seriously than we think, how it was shown that beyond a certain distance from the earth the cosmos is no longer a void but filled with solid crystallized nitrogen. As you can see, things are still so uncertain today that such a view is quite possible. Well, of course that is not the case either but we can nevertheless see from these things the superficial nature of the assumptions which have been made from observation. Because today a person can decide one fine day to imagine that we live here like in an emptied out space which has the slightly solidified earth at the centre and around that the solidified nitrogen which gives us the impression of the starry sky. That is of course also nonsense, but in my view it is indeed the case that people can truly imagine all kinds of things, which accord with external information, about the real make-up of the cosmos. Well it is in fact the case that this report about the crystallized nitrogen might well be an April fool's joke but many people will believe it. It is almost no more stupid to believe such a report than it is to adhere to what is generally assumed to be the case today. And it is brutal materialism to adopt the general assumptions of today. Because in reality the cosmos acts like a hollow sphere and as if forces were entering everywhere from the periphery. It is indeed true that we are dealing with formations which are firmly configured in themselves from outside in, and which can only be modified, differentiated in accordance with the stars so that we already have an original picture of what, in turn, goes on inside us in the configuration of the visible stars. Thus we come to an imagination through this conception showing the human head.

Now, having observed the human head, look at the bird, the way the bird is built. We look at the way the bird is built, and specifically its skeleton, in the wrong way if we simply compare it with a whole human being or a whole animal. You can really only compare the way the bird is built, if you want to compare it at all, with the human head. We have to imagine that we have a modified bird structure in the human head and that the bird has the rest of its body as short appendages in a variety of ways. The legs are always atrophied in birds.

Now imagine the drop formed in such a way that you stretch it into a cylinder. [See Plate 18] If you extend the drop into a cylinder and imagine that what has been differentiated into the head from out of the cosmos remains, but that it continues to be modified in a great variety of

ways because you have extended it into a cylinder, then you have the
torso part of the human being. In order to imagine the torso part of the
human being we have to think of the calotte as atrophied. But then you
have to imagine that when you have the cylinder and invaginate it here,
then you have the third stage. Then you have the limb part of the
human being. It is, however, the case that you first get the limb part of
the human being such that you get what I have drawn here in the arms.
So you have to imagine that you extend and in that way first get the
arms and that the second extension is formed through a second image
being created from inside which originates from the moon. But ignore
the arms for the sake of simplicity. So you go from the sphere to an
extension and then to invagination. If you become used to creating
images in this way through extension and invagination, you are at the
beginning of what you really require to familiarize the soul with
working in the imaginative realm. Because all organized life really
consists of extension and invagination. And just consider how wonderful
that is.

So think that I imagine a sphere and then an extended sphere. That is
the extension upwards caused by the surroundings. If you think here of
the earth with its forces as the counter-image of the surroundings, then
you have the earth below human beings as the thing which invaginates
them. Towards the top, the cosmos extends; towards the bottom, the
earth invaginates. So that you have the image fetched out of the cosmos
and the human being invaginated by the earth. So you can now,
through imagination, answer the question: what would happen if the
earth were not below you and the starry heavens above you? So if you
want to develop imaginations, you never just restrict yourself to
remodelling the human being like this but you have to become used to
seeing all of the cosmos as a whole in the transition from the solid to the
fluid and gradually to imagine less fixed, sharp contours. The fluid is
always fighting against the solid and attempting to integrate it into the
flow, the stream of the whole cosmos. And that is how you get to seeing
such extension and invagination everywhere. You get to seeking the
counter-images everywhere.

As you know, in embryology we never have any indication as to why
things develop the way they do. Embryologists start with the egg cell,

proceed to the cell cluster, see that invagination suddenly occurs and the gastrula is created. That, too, you must imagine as the opportunity being created for the cosmos to work on the one hand, where we have the surface, and that the earth can work where there is invagination [Rudolf Steiner draws, see Plate 19]

Take an epidermal cell that is located near the surface. This is something you have everywhere. There is now a cell close to the surface. The earth principle, which causes invagination, continues its influence in the human being. And so these earth principles are also continuing to be active everywhere. Because of this there is always a tendency to direct the fluid principle in the human being so that it always moves on in this way and an invagination follows. Invagination—pushing in more—invagination—pushing in more—it goes into all kinds of directions. Now imagine something fluid in motion which solidifies. Then look at any organ from this perspective. You can see how it has rigidified, solidified, become invaginated everywhere and on the other hand notice how it is everted. And so you get to the shape of the organs and to a view of how the forces work from all different sides; and you can trace all these organs back to a single form. You only have to be clear that you must start from a very specific point, from the sculptural element. Now you have already pointed out that the forms should be understood through sculpting. But try actually creating a feeling of that for yourselves with a malleable, soft material, taking the material here, on one side, and pushing the clay in that direction with the other hand. Then try and see what develops. You will get a feeling that empty space is pure nonsense. Space is differentiated everywhere by its forces and in this way you will gradually learn to understand all that is sculptural.

Now if you want to understand the human being in sculptural terms you also of course have to be able to go to extremes. I can begin by imagining the sphere here. I imagine that the sphere is expanded on the one side and invaginated on the other. But now imagine that you go further and invaginate here so far that it goes beyond the expanded part. Then you get this kind of structure, indeed, two structures. But now think further that these structures are not just at work on the one side. Imagine you expand, invaginate—expand, invaginate—then an additional invagination from below and expansion upwards, then, if you do that three times, you get the three-dimensional form of the two lungs. In this way you can gradually obtain a view of how the whole of the human being is inwardly connected with such forces and then you move on to the following.

That is a very important idea, the pathological and therapeutic significance of which will only become apparent when the book which Dr Wegman is editing appears.[55] The relationship between the finished organ and organ function will become clear there for the first time. Take organ function. Organ function is constant fluctuation which is kept in a fluid state. The same thing that has completed the organ also produces its activity so that we can say: what is the movement of the juices in the stomach? It is the same thing kept in a fluid state as what the stomach itself is in its solid state. Think of it as frozen movement of the juices, then you have the stomach itself. If that were not the case, it would not be possible at all to cure any organ. You cannot act on the solid organ, only on the fluctuating organ.

Silicic acid acts in the same way as the human kidneys. If similarly I administer silicic acid in Equisetum to a person, I establish a phantom kidney in the area where his kidneys are. This phantom then replaces the astral activity in that location. The latter pushes out the old kidney substance and allows new kidney substance to be formed from out of what is in flow, as also happens in any case after about seven to eight years. The whole business is speeded up by generating such a phantom. We have to understand that everywhere where there is an organ we also constantly have such organ-forming activity and this always solidifies into the organ. That is how you get into the fluid human being.

But then there is still another thing. Then you have to be able to advance to the idea: when I look at the solid human being, I get those nice little pictures in the anatomy books. After all, what we see there is only ten per cent of the human being. That's just how it is. As long as I look at those fixed contours in the human being, then liver = liver, lung = lung, stomach = stomach. But if I then move over to the fluid human being, I can find how this fluid stream is particularly concentrated in, let us say, the liver, and is occupied with building a liver out of the fluid. But each organ always wants to become the whole human being. In the fluid human being that is in fact present as a tendency in each organ so that we have to imagine the following: if I remove the liver it remains a liver, but if I were to take out the fluid out of which the liver is formed, it would have the tendency to become the whole human being. That is what you have to imagine in your imagination: on the one hand the tendency to take on contours, on the other hand to penetrate everything everywhere.

That is simply how it is if we are serious about such things. The meditation formulas contain the beginnings for you to be able gradually to tell yourself the things I am telling you. Everything contains the beginnings to get into the imagination itself. Anyone who starts to meditate has great inner pleasure in meditating to begin with. But at a certain point, when the matter begins to become serious, something rebels because the matter becomes incredibly complicated. If we fail to approach meditation with exceptional seriousness, then we are in the same position as someone who is seeking Lucifer but receives an image of Ahriman. Then the effect of meditation is such that we get the opposite of what we are striving for. The person who seeks Ahriman is given an image of Lucifer. That is the problem. People lose patience and don't stick with it. It is not about time but about the intensive application of patience. Then five minutes can, under certain circumstances, be a long time for meditation. But whether we lose patience in six months or five minutes comes to the same thing. You must have the patience and then you will see how you begin to understand things and how you can move from the solid human being to the fluid human being.

But then you need the musical principle when you move to the aeriform human being. In that situation you have to understand the respiratory processes and if you really meditate then you will become aware of your breathing. The astral, aeriform human being takes shape inwardly. And, you see, then you have to develop a sense for the following: human beings actually go through the world without any self-knowledge. Now they learn to sense themselves, sense themselves with their breathing. If we are in the habit of thinking mathematically or quantitatively, one of the things that occurs at the very beginning is that it suddenly occurs to us to say: am I three halves? You get the feeling as if you were three halves. Why is that so? It is so because we begin to sense through the breathing that on the one side we have a lung divided into three lobes and on the other side one divided into two lobes. And so in this way, by experiencing the inner structures as proportions, we can rise to the astral and aeriform.

And if we can listen very precisely to ourselves in speaking, that is the way to study the I-organization properly. You can also find the I-organization—at first through meditation and then rising to a real understanding—by taking a mammal, say a dog, a skeleton, and studying first the posterior part and then the anterior part very intensively. The one is just the modification of the other. Then you have to progress to the cosmic and imagine the posterior form as having been created by the moon forces and the anterior form by the sun forces. And thus you have to imagine how the sun looks at the moon and then you have the posterior part of the animal in the moon side and the anterior part of the animal in the sun side. And then you have to think of the modification of sun and moon leading to upright posture in human beings and thus you obtain the transformation. The whole matter is relocated by one level and that is another way to reach the I-organization. But this is how you have to proceed: the spatial has to disappear in the sculptural, the sculptural in the musical and the musical in what is meaningful.

If you proceed in this way, you are looking at it from a general perspective and that is actually the healthier way because otherwise you end up in total confusion. You do have to start from these principles and not from the details.

MEDITATION

Preparation: How do I find the good?

1. Can I think the good?

   I cannot think the good.
   Thinking is taken care of by my etheric body.
   My etheric body works in the fluids of the physical body.
   So I will not find the good in the fluids of my physical body.

2. Can I feel the good?

   I can feel the good; but it is not there through me when I only feel it.
   Feeling is taken care of by my astral body.
   My astral body works in the aeriform parts of my body.
   So I will not find the good existing through me in the aeriform parts
   of the body.

3. Can I will the good?

   I can will the good.
   The will is taken care of by my I.
   My I works in the warmth ether of my physical body.
   So I can physically realize the good in warmth.

   I feel my humanity in my warmth.

1. I feel light in my warmth.

   (Ensure that this feeling of light occurs in the region where the
   physical heart is located.)

2. I feel the substance of the world resound in my warmth.

(Ensure that this particular feeling of sound goes from the abdomen to the head but also spreads to the whole of the physical body.)

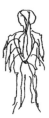

3. I feel in my head cosmic life stirring in my warmth.

(Ensure that the particular feeling of life spreads from the head to the whole of the physical body)

For Helene von Grunelius, autumn 1923

NOTES

Text sources: The lectures in both the courses included in this volume were recorded in shorthand by course participants. With the exception of a number of shorthand notes from the Easter course by Lilly Kolisko, there are no other relevant original shorthand notes in the archives. The textual basis for the publication of the courses is a typed copy which was prepared by unnamed course participants on the basis of their shorthand notes. This copy was neither checked nor authorized by Rudolf Steiner. It was not printed during his lifetime but various additional copies of the transcript were given to interested physicians and students by the leadership of the Medical Section of the School of Spiritual Science. In 1944, the Easter course, edited by Hans W. Zbinden, was published by the Medical Section 'with kind permission of Mrs Steiner'. Hans W. Zbinden was also responsible for the publication of the two courses within the *Gesamtausgabe* (complete edition).

The text was revised for inconsistencies and ambiguous passages in the fourth edition of 2003. The rest are mainly corrections of punctuation and, in some cases, small changes in sentence structure to improve the clarity of the printed text, as the expressiveness of the voice and gestures are not available to aid comprehension. Reference could also be made to Lilly Kolisko's shorthand note in the Easter course. In a few cases, words were inserted which appeared necessary to assist meaning.

The blackboard drawings: The drawings made and texts written on the blackboard covered in black paper in the course of the lectures have been preserved with the exception of the drawings for the lecture of 5 January 1924. They have been published at the end of this volume and in volume XXIII of the series *Rudolf Steiner—Wandtafelzeichnungen zum Vortragswerk* (Rudolf Steiner—Blackboard drawings for the lectures). The black and white drawings by Hedwig Frey inserted in the text in previous editions attempt to reproduce the progression in which the blackboard drawings were created. They have been inserted at the relevant place in the text to the extent that this could be replicated. The original blackboard drawings are referred to in square brackets.

1. It is not clear what lecture is referred to here. Cf. the Stuttgart lecture of 2 March 1920 in *Geisteswissenschaftliche Impulse zur Entwicklung der Physik. Zweiter Naturwissenschaftlicher Kurs: Die Wärme auf der Grenze positiver und negativer Materialität*, GA 321.

2. Lecture of 22 December 1923 in *Mensch und Welt. Das Wirken des Geistes in der Natur. Über die Bienen*, GA 351.

3. The procedure described by Rudolf Steiner here is set out as follows in the Brockhaus encyclopaedia of 1894: 'The caprification of the fig has been well

known since ancient times. Because there is a small gall wasp, the fig wasp (*Cynips psenes* L.), which taps the fig of the wild-growing tree to lay its eggs in it. As a result the wild fig becomes much larger and juicier and also contains more sugar than would otherwise be the case. Therefore tapped wild figs have been hung on the branches of cultivated fig trees since as long ago as antiquity to have their fruit also tapped by the hatching wasps, a process which is now used in all countries where fig trees are cultivated as fruit trees; it is called caprification because the wild fig tree was called Caprificus.'

4. Albert Einstein (1879–1955): 'The principle of relativity', lecture given at the meeting of the Naturforschende Gesellschaft in Zurich on 16 January 1911 entitled 'The Theory of Relativity', published in slightly amended form in *Vierteljahresschrift der Naturforschenden Gesellschaft in Zurich*, volume 36, 1911, pp. 1–14. Cf. also Rudolf Steiner, *Die Rätsel der Philosophy*, GA 18, pp. 590ff.

5. Cf. the lecture of 1 December 1923 in *Mensch und Welt. Das Wirken des Geistes in der Natur. Über die Bienen*, GA 351.

6. Hermann von Helmholtz (1821–94), *Die Lehre von den Tonempfindungen* (On the Sensations of Tone), Brunswick 1892, fifth edition 1896.

7. Cf. the lecture of 22 March 1920 in *Geisteswissenschaft und Medizin*, GA 312.

8. On this little-known phenomenon cf. Bethe-Bermann-Embden, *Handbuch der normalen und pathologischen Physiologie*, volume II, 1928, pp. 196f.

9. The *Handwörterbuch der Naturwissenschaften* of 1912 notes 71 elements in the periodic system.

10. Archimedes, *c.* 287–212 BC. Most important mathematician and engineer of antiquity. Discovered hydrostatic buoyancy and studied the rules of leverage.

11. The Gleno dam in northern Italy failed on 1 December 1923. Cf. Leopold Müller, 'Ein Hinweis Rudolf Steiners zur Sicherung von Talsperren' in *Mitteilungen aus der anthroposophischen Arbeit in Deutschland*, volume 18, issue 4, Christmas 1964.

12. Dr Rudolf Steiner/Dr Ita Wegman, *Grundlegendes für eine Erweiterung der Heilkunst nach geisteswissenschaftlichen Erkenntnissen*, GA 27.
    Ita Wegman, Dr med. (Java 1867–1943 Arlesheim), member since approx. 1903, medical studies in Zurich. Founded the Clinical Therapeutic Institute in Arlesheim which gave rise to intensive collaboration with Rudolf Steiner in the medical field. 1922–24 member of the administrative board of Internationale Laboratorien AG in Arlesheim. 1922–23 member of the closer working group at the Goetheanum. Christmas 1923–35 secretary of the executive council of the General Anthroposophical Society and head of the Medical Section. 1924–25 physician in charge of Rudolf Steiner's treatment.

13. The period starting in about 1840. It built on names including Skoda, Oppolzer, Hebra.

14. 1821–1902, physician and anthropologist, professor of pathological anatomy and cellular pathology.

15. Philippus Aureolus Paracelsus Theophrastus Bombastus von Hohenheim (Einsiedeln 1493–1541 Salzburg). Naturalist, physician and philosopher. 1526–28 city physician and ordinary professor at the University of Basel. Following disputes with the municipal authorities and the medical faculty led an unsettled life in many towns in southern Germany, frequently in great

outer poverty. During this period he composed his great medical and alchemical writings.

16. Youngest epoch of the Permian age. The Rotliegendes rocks were created by continental sedimentation, i.e. conglomerates of sand and clays and volcanic rocks of all sorts collected in the lowland basins in the dry, hot climate. The common but not uniform red colouring comes from haematite, trivalent iron. The name originates from copper shale mining and describes the second layer under the mined mineral; the first is the Weißliegendes. It is essentially only used for its occurrence in Germany, where it surfaces mainly in the area of Chemnitz-Zwickau, Halle, the eastern Harz, Kyffhäuser, Magdeburg, but also in the Saarland and Nahe region.

17. In his autobiography, Rudolf Steiner describes his encounter with a physician who used to walk from Wiener-Neustadt to Neudörfl to care for his patients there. In the book he does not, however, refer to his nature studies but says that the physician revealed the world of German literature to him. It is nevertheless possible that this is one and the same person. Cf. *Mein Lebensgang*, GA 28, pp. 29f.

18. Oil on canvas. 265 × 196 cm. The most famous of Raphael's paintings of the Madonna. It was painted in 1512/13 on commission from Pope Julius II as an altarpiece for the newly built church of the Benedictine monastery in Piacensa, dedicated to Pope Saint Sixtus. The painting hung there relatively unnoticed until the cultured Elector of Saxony and King of Poland, August the Strong, acquired the painting at the start of the eighteenth century for his Dresden collection and it became world famous.

19. Raffaello Sanzio da Urbino (1483–1520). Italian painter. One of the great masters of the Renaissance alongside Leonardo da Vinci and Michelangelo Buonarroti.

20. Ernst Florens Friedrich Chladni (1756–1827). One of the main founders of scientific acoustics. Works: *Entdeckungen über die Theorie des Klangs*, Leipzig 1787, *Akustik*, Leipzig 1802.

21. *Knowledge of the Higher Worlds. How is it achieved?* (1904/05), GA 10.

22. This is likely to have been Kurt Magerstädt and his friends because Magerstädt describes in his reminiscences about Rudolf Steiner how he had chosen the topic of iris diagnosis for his doctoral thesis. He was also interested in palmistry and graphology. Cf. *Wir erlebten Rudolf Steiner* (ed. Krück von Poturzyn), Stuttgart 1956.

23. *The Philosophy of Freedom* (1894), GA 4.

24. 'What is natural is not shameful', saying of the Cynics.

25. The following words of thanks were spoken by Mr van Deventer at the end of the course: 'If I may say a few words on behalf of the members gathered here to thank Dr Steiner and Dr Wegman for what we were privileged to receive here. A feeling arose in our breast through what Dr Steiner gave us in these days, and this feeling was as if our limbs were stretched and our head lifted. We felt that it might after all be possible for us on earth as weak human beings—we felt it as a certainty, that it is possible—to become healers. We stand here with this burning feeling in our hearts, but also in humility. We do not know whether our destiny permits us, and the

extent to which it permits us to unite ourselves with what desires to flow from the Goetheanum for humanity. There are no words to describe what we were privileged to receive as esoteric content, and our feelings, too, are perhaps inadequate. So all that it seems appropriate for us to do is to have the intent.'

26. Cf. pp. xxxff.

27. 1902–92. Studied in Hamburg, Freiburg and Basel. Spent many years in senior positions in Hamburg hospitals, surgeon, ran anthroposophical study groups with students on a private basis.

28. Gautama Buddha (the Enlightened One), *c.* 560–480 BC.

29. Dr med., 1893–1981. Worked from 1925 to 1934 at the Ita Wegman Clinic, mainly as an ophthalmologist. From 1928 to 1971 she had her own practice in Freiburg im Breisgau, Germany, and developed a specific anthroposophical ophthalmology and eurythmy. She returned to Dornach in 1971 and continued to work as a physician to a reduced extent until her death.

30. *Occult Science: An Outline* (1910), GA 113.

31. Elemental hydrogen, like oxygen and nitrogen, always occurs in diatomic form in the air, i.e. H_2, O_2 and N_2

32. Lilly Kolisko (Vienna 1889–1976 Gloucester). Laboratory technician at the Biological Institute at the Goetheanum which was located in Stuttgart. Rudolf Steiner very much appreciated her meticulous work.

33. Lilly Kolisko, *Milzfunktion und Plättchenfrage*, Stuttgart 1922.

34. 1897–1936. As a medical student she was involved in bringing about the two courses for young physicians. In his obituary on Helene von Grunelius, who died at the age of 39 and who only worked for a few years as a physician, the Vienna physician Norbert Glas reports about that time: 'Then the Easter course came. It seemed to me that Rudolf Steiner expected more of us than we were able to bring. He had given us instructions and probably hoped that everything had already properly developed in us. (At least that's how I saw it.) But many of us had probably not advanced as far as we might have done and so Rudolf Steiner opened the Easter course in such a way that it would have been possible for us to ask the right questions of him. He was probably concerned to find a resolution to the problems which had arisen from our work with the Christmas course. But we did not ask many questions in that respect. At that point our friend Helene tossed in a bombshell when she told Dr Steiner how his many indications and instructions made one feel almost despondent. We were annoyed with her—and yet her honesty was admirable.' Quoted from Peter Selg (ed.), *Anthroposophische Ärzte. Lebens- und Arbeitswege im 20. Jahrhundert*, Dornach 2000, p. 229.

35. In the course of the re-founding of the Anthroposophical Society at the Christmas conference of 1923, the esoteric work was also to be placed on a new footing in the form of a three-stage esoteric school. This did not get beyond the establishment of the First Class of this school, comprising 19 lessons. They contain a wealth of meditations. These texts have been published as *Esoterische Unterweisungen für die erste Klasse der Freien Hochschule für Geisteswissenschaft am Goetheanum 1924*, GA 270.

36. *Die Konstitution der Allgemeinen Anthroposophischen Gesellschaft und der Freien*

Hochschule für Geisteswissenschaft. Der Wiederaufbau des Goetheanums 1924–1925, GA 260a.

37. Dr med. Haakon Haakonsen (1881–1933), worked as a general practitioner in Oslo, 1910 member of the Theosophical Society, from 1920 Vidar branch of the Anthroposophical Society.

38. Johann Gottlieb Fichte, 1762–1814. Cf. 'Episode über unser Zeitalter, aus einem republikanischen Schriftsteller', Politisches Fragment, in *Johann Gottlieb Fichtes sämmtliche Werke*, edited by I.H. Fichte, Seventh Volume, Berlin 1846. The quote says a little less extremely: 'As soon as they were older than 30, we might wish for their honour and the benefit of the world that they should die because from then on they would only live to the detriment of themselves and their surroundings.'

39. Cf. *Die Geheimwissenschaft im Umriss*, GA 13, pp. 241f.

40. John Amos Comenius, 1592–1670. Educator and bishop of the Bohemian Brethren, a religious community which had its origins in the Hussite movement and separated completely from the Catholic Church in 1467. Comenius was the last bishop of this older community, which was dissolved during his lifetime but was then re-established by Count Zinzendorf in Herrnhut.

41. Julia Bort, Dr med., 1896–1955, intensively studied eurythmy therapy at the time, was called to work in the Medical Section in 1924 and was subsequently active in curative education.

42. Cf. *Esoterische Betrachtungen karmischer Zusammenhänge*, Volumes I and II, GA 235 and 236.

43. Charlemagne, 742–814. King of the Franks from 768. Was the first German ruler to be crowned Roman Emperor (in Rome by Pope Leo III in 800). He conquered the Saxons, Lombards and Bavarians.

44. 766–809.

45. 1561–1626. English statesman, philosopher, humanist and physician. Creator of empiricism, considered the investigation of natural science to be the only source of certain knowledge.

46. Cf. *Geisteswissenschaft und Medizin* (20 lectures, Dornach 1920), GA 312.

47. 460–377 BC. Greek physician. He was considered to be the greatest physician even in antiquity. The compendium of Greek knowledge about medicine from the fifth and sixth centuries is called the Hippocratic Corpus after him.

48. *c*. 570–632, founder of Islam.

49. Particularly in the lecture of 12 October 1923 in *Das Miterleben des Jahreslaufes in vier kosmischen Imaginationen* (six lectures Dornach/Stuttgart 1923), GA 229.

50. *Truth and Knowledge. Introduction to The Philosophy of Freedom* (1882), GA 3.

51. Margarete Bockholt, Dr med., 1894–1973, at that time an assistant physician at the Clinical and Therapeutic Institute in Arlesheim, worked intensively with eurythmy therapy. In 1955 was appointed to the leadership of the Medical Section at the Goetheanum. From 1963 member of the executive council of the General Anthroposophical Society.

52. The first and only newsletter which appeared during Rudolf Steiner's lifetime.

53. This refers to the so-called warmth meditation which Rudolf Steiner initially gave to Helene von Grunelius in the autumn of 1923 and then also to Ita Wegman to be passed on to physicians. See pp. 240f.

54. Cf. the group sculpture of *The Representative of Humanity between Lucifer and Ahriman*. Rudolf Steiner worked on the 9.5-metre-high wooden group from 1917 to 1924. It was originally intended to stand in a central position under the small cupola of the first Goetheanum but was not yet finished when the Goetheanum burned down during the night of New Year's Eve 1922/1923.
55. See note 12.

RUDOLF STEINER'S COLLECTED WORKS

The German Edition of Rudolf Steiner's Collected Works (the *Gesamtausgabe* [GA] published by Rudolf Steiner Verlag, Dornach, Switzerland) presently runs to 354 titles, organized either by type of work (written or spoken), chronology, audience (public or other), or subject (education, art, etc.). For ease of comparison, the Collected Works in English [CW] follows the German organization exactly. A complete listing of the CWs follows with literal translations of the German titles. Other than in the case of the books published in his lifetime, titles were rarely given by Rudolf Steiner himself, and were often provided by the editors of the German editions. The titles in English are not necessarily the same as the German; and, indeed, over the past seventy-five years have frequently been different, with the same book sometimes appearing under different titles.

For ease of identification and to avoid confusion, we suggest that readers looking for a title should do so by CW number. Because the work of creating the Collected Works of Rudolf Steiner is an ongoing process, with new titles being published every year, we have not indicated in this listing which books are presently available. To find out what titles in the Collected Works are currently in print, please check our website at www.rudolfsteinerpress.com (or www.steinerbooks.org for US readers).

Written Work

CW 1	Goethe: Natural-Scientific Writings, Introduction, with Footnotes and Explanations in the text by Rudolf Steiner
CW 2	Outlines of an Epistemology of the Goethean World View, with Special Consideration of Schiller
CW 3	Truth and Science
CW 4	The Philosophy of Freedom
CW 4a	Documents to 'The Philosophy of Freedom'
CW 5	Friedrich Nietzsche, A Fighter against His Own Time
CW 6	Goethe's Worldview
CW 6a	Now in CW 30
CW 7	Mysticism at the Dawn of Modern Spiritual Life and Its Relationship with Modern Worldviews
CW 8	Christianity as Mystical Fact and the Mysteries of Antiquity
CW 9	Theosophy: An Introduction into Supersensible World Knowledge and Human Purpose
CW 10	How Does One Attain Knowledge of Higher Worlds?
CW 11	From the Akasha-Chronicle

Public Lectures

CW 51	On Philosophy, History and Literature
CW 52	Spiritual Teachings Concerning the Soul and Observation of the World
CW 53	The Origin and Goal of the Human Being
CW 54	The Riddles of the World and Anthroposophy
CW 55	Knowledge of the Supersensible in Our Times and Its Meaning for Life Today
CW 56	Knowledge of the Soul and of the Spirit
CW 57	Where and How Does One Find the Spirit?
CW 58	The Metamorphoses of the Soul Life. Paths of Soul Experiences: Part One
CW 59	The Metamorphoses of the Soul Life. Paths of Soul Experiences: Part Two
CW 60	The Answers of Spiritual Science to the Biggest Questions of Existence
CW 61	Human History in the Light of Spiritual Research
CW 62	Results of Spiritual Research
CW 63	Spiritual Science as a Treasure for Life
CW 64	Out of Destiny-Burdened Times
CW 65	Out of Central European Spiritual Life
CW 66	Spirit and Matter, Life and Death
CW 67	The Eternal in the Human Soul. Immortality and Freedom
CW 68	Public lectures in various cities, 1906–1918
CW 69	Public lectures in various cities, 1906–1918
CW 70	Public lectures in various cities, 1906–1918
CW 71	Public lectures in various cities, 1906–1918
CW 72	Freedom—Immortality—Social Life
CW 73	The Supplementing of the Modern Sciences through Anthroposophy
CW 73a	Specialized Fields of Knowledge and Anthroposophy
CW 74	The Philosophy of Thomas Aquinas
CW 75	Public lectures in various cities, 1906–1918
CW 76	The Fructifying Effect of Anthroposophy on Specialized Fields
CW 77a	The Task of Anthroposophy in Relation to Science and Life: The Darmstadt College Course
CW 77b	Art and Anthroposophy. The Goetheanum-Impulse
CW 78	Anthroposophy, Its Roots of Knowledge and Fruits for Life
CW 79	The Reality of the Higher Worlds
CW 80	Public lectures in various cities, 1922
CW 81	Renewal-Impulses for Culture and Science—Berlin College Course
CW 82	So that the Human Being Can Become a Complete Human Being
CW 83	Western and Eastern World-Contrast. Paths to Understanding It through Anthroposophy
CW 84	What Did the Goetheanum Intend and What Should Anthroposophy Do?

Lectures to the Members of the Anthroposophical Society

CW 240 Esoteric Observations of Karmic Relationships in 6 Volumes, Vol. 6
CW 243 The Consciousness of the Initiate
CW 245 Instructions for an Esoteric Schooling
CW 250 The Building-Up of the Anthroposophical Society. From the Beginning to the Outbreak of the First World War
CW 251 The History of the Goetheanum Building-Association
CW 252 Life in the Anthroposophical Society from the First World War to the Burning of the First Goetheanum
CW 253 The Problems of Living Together in the Anthroposophical Society. On the Dornach Crisis of 1915. With Highlights on Swedenborg's Clairvoyance, the Views of Freudian Psychoanalysts, and the Concept of Love in Relation to Mysticism
CW 254 The Occult Movement in the 19th Century and Its Relationship to World Culture. Significant Points from the Exoteric Cultural Life around the Middle of the 19th Century
CW 255 Rudolf Steiner during the First World War
CW 255a Anthroposophy and the Reformation of Society. On the History of the Threefold Movement
CW 255b Anthroposophy and Its Opponents, 1919–1921
CW 256 How Can the Anthroposophical Movement Be Financed?
CW 256a Futurum, Inc. / International Laboratories, Inc.
CW 256b The Coming Day, Inc.
CW 257 Anthroposophical Community-Building
CW 258 The History of and Conditions for the Anthroposophical Movement in Relationship to the Anthroposophical Society. A Stimulus to Self-Contemplation
CW 259 The Year of Destiny 1923 in the History of the Anthroposophical Society. From the Burning of the Goetheanum to the Christmas Conference
CW 260 The Christmas Conference for the Founding of the General Anthroposophical Society
CW 260a The Constitution of the General Anthroposophical Society and the School for Spiritual Science. The Rebuilding of the Goetheanum
CW 261 Our Dead. Addresses, Words of Remembrance, and Meditative Verses, 1906–1924
CW 262 Rudolf Steiner and Marie Steiner-von Sivers: Correspondence and Documents, 1901–1925
CW 263/1 Rudolf Steiner and Edith Maryon: Correspondence: Letters, Verses, Sketches, 1912–1924
CW 264 On the History and the Contents of the First Section of the Esoteric School from 1904 to 1914. Letters, Newsletters, Documents, Lectures
CW 265 On the History and from the Contents of the Ritual-Knowledge Section of the Esoteric School from 1904 to 1914. Documents, and Lectures from the Years 1906 to 1914, as Well as on New Approaches to Ritual-Knowledge Work in the Years 1921–1924

CW 266/1   From the Contents of the Esoteric Lessons. Volume 1: 1904–1909. Notes from Memory of Participants. Meditation texts from the notes of Rudolf Steiner

CW 266/2   From the Contents of the Esoteric Lessons. Volume 2: 1910–1912. Notes from Memory of Participants

CW 266/3   From the Contents of the Esoteric Lessons. Volume 3: 1913, 1914 and 1920–1923. Notes from Memory of Participants. Meditation texts from the notes of Rudolf Steiner

CW 267   Soul-Exercises: Vol. 1: Exercises with Word and Image Meditations for the Methodological Development of Higher Powers of Knowledge, 1904–1924

CW 268   Soul-Exercises: Vol. 2: Mantric Verses, 1903–1925

CW 269   Ritual Texts for the Celebration of the Free Christian Religious Instruction. The Collected Verses for Teachers and Students of the Waldorf School

CW 270   Esoteric Instructions for the First Class of the School for Spiritual Science at the Goetheanum 1924, 4 Volumes

CW 271   Art and Knowledge of Art. Foundations of a New Aesthetic

CW 272   Spiritual-Scientific Commentary on Goethe's 'Faust' in Two Volumes. Vol. 1: Faust, the Striving Human Being

CW 273   Spiritual-Scientific Commentary on Goethe's 'Faust' in Two Volumes. Vol. 2: The Faust-Problem

CW 274   Addresses for the Christmas Plays from the Old Folk Traditions

CW 275   Art in the Light of Mystery-Wisdom

CW 276   The Artistic in Its Mission in the World. The Genius of Language. The World of Self-Revealing Radiant Appearances—Anthroposophy and Art. Anthroposophy and Poetry

CW 277   Eurythmy. The Revelation of the Speaking Soul

CW 277a   The Origin and Development of Eurythmy

CW 278   Eurythmy as Visible Song

CW 279   Eurythmy as Visible Speech

CW 280   The Method and Nature of Speech Formation

CW 281   The Art of Recitation and Declamation

CW 282   Speech Formation and Dramatic Art

CW 283   The Nature of Things Musical and the Experience of Tone in the Human Being

CW 284/285   Images of Occult Seals and Pillars. The Munich Congress of Whitsun 1907 and Its Consequences

CW 286   Paths to a New Style of Architecture. 'And the Building Becomes Human'

CW 287   The Building at Dornach as a Symbol of Historical Becoming and an Artistic Transformation Impulse

CW 288   Style-Forms in the Living Organic

CW 289   The Building-Idea of the Goetheanum: Lectures with Slides from the Years 1920–1921

CW 290   The Building-Idea of the Goetheanum: Lectures with Slides from the Years 1920–1921

SIGNIFICANT EVENTS IN THE LIFE OF
RUDOLF STEINER

1829:   June 23: birth of Johann Steiner (1829–1910)—Rudolf Steiner's father—in Geras, Lower Austria.

1834:   May 8: birth of Franciska Blie (1834–1918)—Rudolf Steiner's mother—in Horn, Lower Austria. 'My father and mother were both children of the glorious Lower Austrian forest district north of the Danube.'

1860:   May 16: marriage of Johann Steiner and Franciska Blie.

1861:   February 25: birth of *Rudolf Joseph Lorenz Steiner* in Kraljevec, Croatia, near the border with Hungary, where Johann Steiner works as a telegrapher for the South Austria Railroad. Rudolf Steiner is baptized two days later, February 27, the date usually given as his birthday.

1862:   Summer: the family moves to Mödling, Lower Austria.

1863:   The family moves to Pottschach, Lower Austria, near the Styrian border, where Johann Steiner becomes stationmaster. 'The view stretched to the mountains ... majestic peaks in the distance and the sweet charm of nature in the immediate surroundings.'

1864:   November 15: birth of Rudolf Steiner's sister, Leopoldine (d. November 1, 1927). She will become a seamstress and live with her parents for the rest of her life.

1866:   July 28: birth of Rudolf Steiner's deaf-mute brother, Gustav (d. May 1, 1941).

1867:   Rudolf Steiner enters the village school. Following a disagreement between his father and the schoolmaster, whose wife falsely accused the boy of causing a commotion, Rudolf Steiner is taken out of school and taught at home.

1868:   A critical experience. Unknown to the family, an aunt dies in a distant town. Sitting in the station waiting room, Rudolf Steiner sees her 'form,' which speaks to him, asking for help. 'Beginning with this experience, a new soul life began in the boy, one in which not only the outer trees and mountains spoke to him, but also the worlds that lay behind them. From this moment on, the boy began to live with the spirits of nature...'

1869:   The family moves to the peaceful, rural village of Neudorfl, near Wiener-Neustadt in present-day Austria. Rudolf Steiner attends the village school. Because of the 'unorthodoxy' of his writing and spelling, he has to do 'extra lessons.'

1870:   Through a book lent to him by his tutor, he discovers geometry: 'To grasp something purely in the spirit brought me inner happiness. I know that I first learned happiness through geometry.' The same tutor allows him to draw, while other students still struggle with their reading and writing. 'An artistic element' thus enters his education.

1871: Though his parents are not religious, Rudolf Steiner becomes a 'church child,' a favorite of the priest, who was 'an exceptional character.' 'Up to the age of ten or eleven, among those I came to know, he was far and away the most significant.' Among other things, he introduces Steiner to Copernican, heliocentric cosmology. As an altar boy, Rudolf Steiner serves at Masses, funerals, and Corpus Christi processions. At year's end, after an incident in which he escapes a thrashing, his father forbids him to go to church.

1872: Rudolf Steiner transfers to grammar school in Wiener-Neustadt, a five-mile walk from home, which must be done in all weathers.

1873–75: Through his teachers and on his own, Rudolf Steiner has many wonderful experiences with science and mathematics. Outside school, he teaches himself analytic geometry, trigonometry, differential equations, and calculus.

1876: Rudolf Steiner begins tutoring other students. He learns bookbinding from his father. He also teaches himself stenography.

1877: Rudolf Steiner discovers Kant's *Critique of Pure Reason*, which he reads and rereads. He also discovers and reads von Rotteck's *World History*.

1878: He studies extensively in contemporary psychology and philosophy.

1879: Rudolf Steiner graduates from high school with honors. His father is transferred to Inzersdorf, near Vienna. He uses his first visit to Vienna 'to purchase a great number of philosophy books'—Kant, Fichte, Schelling, and Hegel, as well as numerous histories of philosophy. His aim: to find a path from the 'I' to nature.

October 1879–1883: Rudolf Steiner attends the Technical College in Vienna—to study mathematics, chemistry, physics, mineralogy, botany, zoology, biology, geology, and mechanics—with a scholarship. He also attends lectures in history and literature, while avidly reading philosophy on his own. His two favorite professors are Karl Julius Schröer (German language and literature) and Edmund Reitlinger (physics). He also audits lectures by Robert Zimmerman on aesthetics and Franz Brentano on philosophy. During this year he begins his friendship with Moritz Zitter (1861–1921), who will help support him financially when he is in Berlin.

1880: Rudolf Steiner attends lectures on Schiller and Goethe by Karl Julius Schröer, who becomes his mentor. Also 'through a remarkable combination of circumstances,' he meets Felix Koguzki, a 'herb gatherer' and healer, who could 'see deeply into the secrets of nature.' Rudolf Steiner will meet and study with this 'emissary of the Master' throughout his time in Vienna.

1881: January: '... I didn't sleep a wink. I was busy with philosophical problems until about 12:30 a.m. Then, finally, I threw myself down on my couch. All my striving during the previous year had been to research whether the following statement by Schelling was true or not: *Within everyone dwells a secret, marvelous capacity to draw back from the stream of time—out of the self clothed in all that comes to us from outside—into our innermost being and there, in the immutable form of the Eternal, to look into ourselves.* I believe, and I am still quite certain of it, that I discovered this capacity in myself; I had long had an inkling of it. Now the whole of idealist philosophy stood before me in modified form. What's a sleepless night compared to that!'

Rudolf Steiner begins communicating with leading thinkers of the day, who send him books in return, which he reads eagerly.

July: 'I am not one of those who dives into the day like an animal in human form. I pursue a quite specific goal, an idealistic aim—knowledge of the truth! This cannot be done offhandedly. It requires the greatest striving in the world, free of all egotism, and equally of all resignation.'

August: Steiner puts down on paper for the first time thoughts for a 'Philosophy of Freedom.' 'The striving for the absolute: this human yearning is freedom.' He also seeks to outline a 'peasant philosophy,' describing what the worldview of a 'peasant'—one who lives close to the earth and the old ways—really is.

1881–1882: Felix Koguzki, the herb gatherer, reveals himself to be the envoy of another, higher initiatory personality, who instructs Rudolf Steiner to penetrate Fichte's philosophy and to master modern scientific thinking as a preparation for right entry into the spirit. This 'Master' also teaches him the double (evolutionary and involutionary) nature of time.

1882: Through the offices of Karl Julius Schröer, Rudolf Steiner is asked by Joseph Kurschner to edit Goethe's scientific works for the *Deutschen National-Literatur* edition. He writes 'A Possible Critique of Atomistic Concepts' and sends it to Friedrich Theodore Vischer.

1883: Rudolf Steiner completes his college studies and begins work on the Goethe project.

1884: First volume of Goethe's *Scientific Writings* (CW 1) appears (March). He lectures on Goethe and Lessing, and Goethe's approach to science. In July, he enters the household of Ladislaus and Pauline Specht as tutor to the four Specht boys. He will live there until 1890. At this time, he meets Josef Breuer (1842–1925), the coauthor with Sigmund Freud of *Studies in Hysteria*, who is the Specht family doctor.

1885: While continuing to edit Goethe's writings, Rudolf Steiner reads deeply in contemporary philosophy (Edouard von Hartmann, Johannes Volkelt, and Richard Wahle, among others).

1886: May: Rudolf Steiner sends Kurschner the manuscript of *Outlines of Goethe's Theory of Knowledge* (CW 2), which appears in October, and which he sends out widely. He also meets the poet Marie Eugenie Delle Grazie and writes 'Nature and Our Ideals' for her. He attends her salon, where he meets many priests, theologians, and philosophers, who will become his friends. Meanwhile, the director of the Goethe Archive in Weimar requests his collaboration with the *Sophien* edition of Goethe's works, particularly the writings on color.

1887: At the beginning of the year, Rudolf Steiner is very sick. As the year progresses and his health improves, he becomes increasingly 'a man of letters,' lecturing, writing essays, and taking part in Austrian cultural life. In August–September, the second volume of Goethe's *Scientific Writings* appears.

1888: January–July: Rudolf Steiner assumes editorship of the 'German Weekly' (*Deutsche Wochenschrift*). He begins lecturing more intensively, giving, for example, a lecture titled 'Goethe as Father of a New Aesthetics.' He meets and becomes soul friends with Friedrich Eckstein (1861–1939), a vegetarian, philosopher of symbolism, alchemist, and musician, who will introduce him to various spiritual currents (including Theosophy) and with whom he will meditate and interpret esoteric and alchemical texts.

1889: Rudolf Steiner first reads Nietzsche (*Beyond Good and Evil*). He encounters Theosophy again and learns of Madame Blavatsky in the Theosophical circle around Marie Lang (1858–1934). Here he also meets well-known figures of Austrian life, as well as esoteric figures like the occultist Franz Hartman and Karl Leinigen-Billigen (translator of C.G. Harrison's *The Transcendental Universe*). During this period, Steiner first reads A.P. Sinnett's *Esoteric Buddhism* and Mabel Collins's *Light on the Path*. He also begins traveling, visiting Budapest, Weimar, and Berlin (where he meets philosopher Edouard von Hartmann).

1890: Rudolf Steiner finishes volume 3 of Goethe's scientific writings. He begins his doctoral dissertation, which will become *Truth and Science* (CW 3). He also meets the poet and feminist Rosa Mayreder (1858–1938), with whom he can exchange his most intimate thoughts. In September, Rudolf Steiner moves to Weimar to work in the Goethe-Schiller Archive.

1891: Volume 3 of the Kurschner edition of Goethe appears. Meanwhile, Rudolf Steiner edits Goethe's studies in mineralogy and scientific writings for the *Sophien* edition. He meets Ludwig Laistner of the Cotta Publishing Company, who asks for a book on the basic question of metaphysics. From this will result, ultimately, *The Philosophy of Freedom* (CW 4), which will be published not by Cotta but by Emil Felber. In October, Rudolf Steiner takes the oral exam for a doctorate in philosophy, mathematics, and mechanics at Rostock University, receiving his doctorate on the twenty-sixth. In November, he gives his first lecture on Goethe's 'Fairy Tale' in Vienna.

1892: Rudolf Steiner continues work at the Goethe-Schiller Archive and on his *Philosophy of Freedom*. *Truth and Science*, his doctoral dissertation, is published. Steiner undertakes to write introductions to books on Schopenhauer and Jean Paul for Cotta. At year's end, he finds lodging with Anna Eunike, née Schulz (1853–1911), a widow with four daughters and a son. He also develops a friendship with Otto Erich Hartleben (1864–1905) with whom he shares literary interests.

1893: Rudolf Steiner begins his habit of producing many reviews and articles. In March, he gives a lecture titled 'Hypnotism, with Reference to Spiritism.' In September, volume 4 of the Kurschner edition is completed. In November, *The Philosophy of Freedom* appears. This year, too, he meets John Henry Mackay (1864–1933), the anarchist, and Max Stirner, a scholar and biographer.

1894: Rudolf Steiner meets Elisabeth Förster Nietzsche, the philosopher's sister, and begins to read Nietzsche in earnest, beginning with the as yet unpublished *Antichrist*. He also meets Ernst Haeckel (1834–1919). In the fall, he begins to write *Nietzsche, A Fighter against His Time* (CW 5).

1895:   May, *Nietzsche, A Fighter against His Time* appears.

1896:   January 22: Rudolf Steiner sees Friedrich Nietzsche for the first and only time. Moves between the Nietzsche and the Goethe-Schiller Archives, where he completes his work before year's end. He falls out with Elisabeth Förster Nietzsche, thus ending his association with the Nietzsche Archive.

1897:   Rudolf Steiner finishes the manuscript of *Goethe's Worldview* (CW 6). He moves to Berlin with Anna Eunike and begins editorship of the *Magazin für Literatur*. From now on, Steiner will write countless reviews, literary and philosophical articles, and so on. He begins lecturing at the 'Free Literary Society.' In September, he attends the Zionist Congress in Basel. He sides with Dreyfus in the Dreyfus affair.

1898:   Rudolf Steiner is very active as an editor in the political, artistic, and theatrical life of Berlin. He becomes friendly with John Henry Mackay and poet Ludwig Jacobowski (1868–1900). He joins Jacobowski's circle of writers, artists, and scientists—'The Coming Ones' (*Die Kommenden*)— and contributes lectures to the group until 1903. He also lectures at the 'League for College Pedagogy.' He writes an article for Goethe's sesquicentennial, 'Goethe's Secret Revelation,' on the 'Fairy Tale of the Green Snake and the Beautiful Lily.'

1898–99: 'This was a trying time for my soul as I looked at Christianity. . . . I was able to progress only by contemplating, by means of spiritual perception, the evolution of Christianity. . . . Conscious knowledge of real Christianity began to dawn in me around the turn of the century. This seed continued to develop. My soul trial occurred shortly before the beginning of the twentieth century. It was decisive for my soul's development that I stood spiritually before the Mystery of Golgotha in a deep and solemn celebration of knowledge.'

1899:   Rudolf Steiner begins teaching and giving lectures and lecture cycles at the Workers' College, founded by Wilhelm Liebknecht (1826–1900). He will continue to do so until 1904. Writes: *Literature and Spiritual Life in the Nineteenth Century; Individualism in Philosophy*; *Haeckel and His Opponents; Poetry in the Present;* and begins what will become (fifteen years later) *The Riddles of Philosophy* (CW 18). He also meets many artists and writers, including Käthe Kollwitz, Stefan Zweig, and Rainer Maria Rilke. On October 31, he marries Anna Eunike.

1900:   'I thought that the turn of the century must bring humanity a new light. It seemed to me that the separation of human thinking and willing from the spirit had peaked. A turn or reversal of direction in human evolution seemed to me a necessity.' Rudolf Steiner finishes *World and Life Views in the Nineteenth Century* (the second part of what will become *The Riddles of Philosophy*) and dedicates it to Ernst Haeckel. It is published in March. He continues lecturing at *Die Kommenden*, whose leadership he assumes after the death of Jacobowski. Also, he gives the Gutenberg Jubilee lecture before 7,000 typesetters and printers. In September, Rudolf Steiner is invited by Count and Countess Brockdorff to lecture in the Theosophical Library. His first lecture is on Nietzsche. His second lecture is titled 'Goethe's Secret Revelation.' October 6, he begins a lecture cycle on the mystics that will become *Mystics after Modernism* (CW 7). November–December: 'Marie von Sivers appears in the audience. . . .' Also in November, Steiner gives his first lecture at the Giordano Bruno Bund (where he will continue to lecture until May, 1905). He speaks on Bruno and modern Rome, focusing on the importance of the philosophy of Thomas Aquinas as monism.

1901:   In continual financial straits, Rudolf Steiner's early friends Moritz Zitter and Rosa Mayreder help support him. In October, he begins the lecture cycle *Christianity as Mystical Fact* (CW 8) at the Theosophical Library. In November, he gives his first 'Theosophical lecture' on Goethe's 'Fairy Tale' in Hamburg at the invitation of Wilhelm Hubbe-Schleiden. He also attends a gathering to celebrate the founding of the Theosophical Society at Count and Countess Brockdorff's. He gives a lecture cycle, 'From Buddha to Christ,' for the circle of the *Kommenden*. November 17, Marie von Sivers asks Rudolf Steiner if Theosophy needs a Western-Christian spiritual movement (to complement Theosophy's Eastern emphasis). 'The question was posed. Now, following spiritual laws, I could begin to give an answer. . . .' In December, Rudolf Steiner writes his first article for a Theosophical publication. At year's end, the Brockdorffs and possibly Wilhelm Hubbe-Schleiden ask Rudolf Steiner to join the Theosophical Society and undertake the leadership of the German section. Rudolf Steiner agrees, on the condition that Marie von Sivers (then in Italy) work with him.

1902:   Beginning in January, Rudolf Steiner attends the opening of the Workers' School in Spandau with Rosa Luxemberg (1870–1919). January 17, Rudolf Steiner joins the Theosophical Society. In April, he is asked to become general secretary of the German Section of the Theosophical Society, and works on preparations for its founding. In July, he visits London for a Theosophical congress. He meets Bertram Keightly, G.R.S. Mead, A.P. Sinnett, and Annie Besant, among others. In September, *Christianity as Mystical Fact* appears. In October, Rudolf Steiner gives his first public lecture on Theosophy ('Monism and Theosophy') to about three hundred people at the Giordano Bruno Bund. On October 19–21, the German Section of the Theosophical Society has its first meeting; Rudolf Steiner is the general secretary, and Annie Besant attends. Steiner lectures on practical karma studies. On October 23, Annie Besant inducts Rudolf Steiner into the Esoteric School of the Theosophical Society. On October 25, Steiner begins a weekly series of lectures: 'The Field of Theosophy.' During this year, Rudolf Steiner also first meets Ita Wegman (1876–1943), who will become his close collaborator in his final years.

1903:   Rudolf Steiner holds about 300 lectures and seminars. In May, the first issue of the periodical *Luzifer* appears. In June, Rudolf Steiner visits

London for the first meeting of the Federation of the European Sections of the Theosophical Society, where he meets Colonel Olcott. He begins to write *Theosophy* (CW 9).

1904:   Rudolf Steiner continues lecturing at the Workers' College and elsewhere (about 90 lectures), while lecturing intensively all over Germany among Theosophists (about 140 lectures). In February, he meets Carl Unger (1878–1929), who will become a member of the board of the Anthroposophical Society (1913). In March, he meets Michael Bauer (1871–1929), a Christian mystic, who will also be on the board. In May, *Theosophy* appears, with the dedication: 'To the spirit of Giordano Bruno.' Rudolf Steiner and Marie von Sivers visit London for meetings with Annie Besant. June: Rudolf Steiner and Marie von Sivers attend the meeting of the Federation of European Sections of the Theosophical Society in Amsterdam. In July, Steiner begins the articles in *Luzifer-Gnosis* that will become *How to Know Higher Worlds* (CW 10) and *Cosmic Memory* (CW 11). In September, Annie Besant visits Germany. In December, Steiner lectures on Freemasonry. He mentions the High Grade Masonry derived from John Yarker and represented by Theodore Reuss and Karl Kellner as a blank slate 'into which a good image could be placed.'

1905:   This year, Steiner ends his non-Theosophical lecturing activity. Supported by Marie von Sivers, his Theosophical lecturing—both in public and in the Theosophical Society—increases significantly: 'The German Theosophical Movement is of exceptional importance.' Steiner recommends reading, among others, Fichte, Jacob Boehme, and Angelus Silesius. He begins to introduce Christian themes into Theosophy. He also begins to work with doctors (Felix Peipers and Ludwig Noll). In July, he is in London for the Federation of European Sections, where he attends a lecture by Annie Besant: 'I have seldom seen Mrs. Besant speak in so inward and heartfelt a manner....' 'Through Mrs. Besant I have found the way to H.P. Blavatsky.' September to October, he gives a course of thirty-one lectures for a small group of esoteric students. In October, the annual meeting of the German Section of the Theosophical Society, which still remains very small, takes place. Rudolf Steiner reports membership has risen from 121 to 377 members. In November, seeking to establish esoteric 'continuity,' Rudolf Steiner and Marie von Sivers participate in a 'Memphis-Misraim' Masonic ceremony. They pay forty-five marks for membership. 'Yesterday, you saw how little remains of former esoteric institutions.' 'We are dealing only with a "framework"... for the present, nothing lies behind it. The occult powers have completely withdrawn.'

1906:   Expansion of Theosophical work. Rudolf Steiner gives about 245 lectures, only 44 of which take place in Berlin. Cycles are given in Paris, Leipzig, Stuttgart, and Munich. Esoteric work also intensifies. Rudolf Steiner begins writing *An Outline of Esoteric Science* (CW 13). In January, Rudolf Steiner receives permission (a patent) from the Great Orient of the Scottish A & A Thirty-Three Degree Rite of the Order of the Ancient

Freemasons of the Memphis-Misraim Rite to direct a chapter under the name 'Mystica Aeterna.' This will become the 'Cognitive-Ritual Section' (also called 'Misraim Service') of the Esoteric School. (See: *Freemasonry and Ritual Work: The Misraim Service*, CW 265). During this time, Steiner also meets Albert Schweitzer. In May, he is in Paris, where he visits Edouard Schuré. Many Russians attend his lectures (including Konstantin Balmont, Dimitri Mereszkovski, Zinaida Hippius, and Maximilian Woloshin). He attends the General Meeting of the European Federation of the Theosophical Society, at which Col. Olcott is present for the last time. He spends the year's end in Venice and Rome, where he writes and works on his translation of H.P. Blavatsky's *Key to Theosophy*.

1907:   Further expansion of the German Theosophical Movement according to the Rosicrucian directive to 'introduce spirit into the world'—in education, in social questions, in art, and in science. In February, Col. Olcott dies in Adyar. Before he dies, Olcott indicates that 'the Masters' wish Annie Besant to succeed him: much politicking ensues. Rudolf Steiner supports Besant's candidacy. April-May: preparations for the Congress of the Federation of European Sections of the Theosophical Society—the great, watershed Whitsun 'Munich Congress,' attended by Annie Besant and others. Steiner decides to separate Eastern and Western (Christian-Rosicrucian) esoteric schools. He takes his esoteric school out of the Theosophical Society (Besant and Rudolf Steiner are 'in harmony' on this). Steiner makes his first lecture tours to Austria and Hungary. That summer, he is in Italy. In September, he visits Edouard Schuré, who will write the introduction to the French edition of *Christianity as Mystical Fact* in Barr, Alsace. Rudolf Steiner writes the autobiographical statement known as the 'Barr Document.' In *Luzifer-Gnosis*, 'The Education of the Child' appears.

1908:   The movement grows (membership: 1,150). Lecturing expands. Steiner makes his first extended lecture tour to Holland and Scandinavia, as well as visits to Naples and Sicily. Themes: St. John's Gospel, the Apocalypse, Egypt, science, philosophy, and logic. *Luzifer-Gnosis* ceases publication. In Berlin, Marie von Sivers (with Johanna Mücke (1864–1949) forms the *Philosophisch-Theosophisch* (after 1915 *Philosophisch-Anthroposophisch*) *Verlag* to publish Steiner's work. Steiner gives lecture cycles titled *The Gospel of St. John* (CW 103) and *The Apocalypse* (104).

1909:   *An Outline of Esoteric Science* appears. Lecturing and travel continues. Rudolf Steiner's spiritual research expands to include the polarity of Lucifer and Ahriman; the work of great individualities in history; the Maitreya Buddha and the Bodhisattvas; spiritual economy (CW 109); the work of the spiritual hierarchies in heaven and on earth (CW 110). He also deepens and intensifies his research into the Gospels, giving lectures on the Gospel of St. Luke (CW 114) with the first mention of two Jesus children. Meets and becomes friends with Christian Morgenstern (1871–1914). In April, he lays the foundation stone for the Malsch model—the building that will lead to the first Goetheanum. In May, the International Congress of the Federation of European Sections of the

Theosophical Society takes place in Budapest. Rudolf Steiner receives the Subba Row medal for *How to Know Higher Worlds*. During this time, Charles W. Leadbeater discovers Jiddu Krishnamurti (1895–1986) and proclaims him the future 'world teacher,' the bearer of the Maitreya Buddha and the 'reappearing Christ.' In October, Steiner delivers seminal lectures on 'anthroposophy,' which he will try, unsuccessfully, to rework over the next years into the unfinished work, *Anthroposophy (A Fragment)* (CW 45).

1910: New themes: *The Reappearance of Christ in the Etheric* (CW 118); *The Fifth Gospel; The Mission of Folk Souls* (CW 121); *Occult History* (CW 126); the evolving development of etheric cognitive capacities. Rudolf Steiner continues his Gospel research with *The Gospel of St. Matthew* (CW 123). In January, his father dies. In April, he takes a month-long trip to Italy, including Rome, Monte Cassino, and Sicily. He also visits Scandinavia again. July–August, he writes the first mystery drama, *The Portal of Initiation* (CW 14). In November, he gives 'psychosophy' lectures. In December, he submits 'On the Psychological Foundations and Episte-mological Framework of Theosophy' to the International Philosophical Congress in Bologna.

1911: The crisis in the Theosophical Society deepens. In January, 'The Order of the Rising Sun,' which will soon become 'The Order of the Star in the East,' is founded for the coming world teacher, Krishnamurti. At the same time, Marie von Sivers, Rudolf Steiner's coworker, falls ill. Fewer lectures are given, but important new ground is broken. In Prague, in March, Steiner meets Franz Kafka (1883–1924) and Hugo Bergmann (1883-1975). In April, he delivers his paper to the Philosophical Con-gress. He writes the second mystery drama, *The Soul's Probation* (CW 14). Also, while Marie von Sivers is convalescing, Rudolf Steiner begins work on *Calendar 1912/1913*, which will contain the 'Calendar of the Soul' meditations. On March 19, Anna (Eunike) Steiner dies. In September, Rudolf Steiner visits Einsiedeln, birthplace of Paracelsus. In December, Friedrich Rittelmeyer, future founder of the Christian Community, meets Rudolf Steiner. The *Johannes-Bauverein*, the 'building committee,' which would lead to the first Goetheanum (first planned for Munich), is also founded, and a preliminary committee for the founding of an indepen-dent association is created that, in the following year, will become the Anthroposophical Society. Important lecture cycles include *Occult Phy-siology* (CW 128); *Wonders of the World* (CW 129); *From Jesus to Christ* (CW 131). Other themes: esoteric Christianity; Christian Rosenkreutz; the spiritual guidance of humanity; the sense world and the world of the spirit.

1912: Despite the ongoing, now increasing crisis in the Theosophical Society, much is accomplished: *Calendar 1912/1913* is published; eurythmy is created; both the third mystery drama, *The Guardian of the Threshold* (CW 14) and *A Way of Self-Knowledge* (CW 16) are written. New (or renewed) themes included life between death and rebirth and karma and reincarnation. Other lecture cycles: *Spiritual Beings in the Heavenly Bodies and in the Kingdoms of Nature* (CW 136); *The Human Being in the Light of Occultism, Theosophy, and Philosophy* (CW 137); *The Gospel of St. Mark* (CW 139); and *The Bhagavad Gita and the Epistles of Paul* (CW 142). On May 8, Rudolf Steiner celebrates White Lotus Day, H.P. Blavatsky's death day, which he had faithfully observed for the past decade, for the last time. In August, Rudolf Steiner suggests the 'independent association' be called the 'Anthroposophical Society.' In September, the first eurythmy course takes place. In October, Rudolf Steiner declines recognition of a Theosophical Society lodge dedicated to the Star of the East and decides to expel all Theosophical Society members belonging to the order. Also, with Marie von Sivers, he first visits Dornach, near Basel, Switzerland, and they stand on the hill where the Goetheanum will be built. In November, a Theosophical Society lodge is opened by direct mandate from Adyar (Annie Besant). In December, a meeting of the German section occurs at which it is decided that belonging to the Order of the Star of the East is incompatible with membership in the Theosophical Society. December 28: informal founding of the Anthroposophical Society in Berlin.

1913:   Expulsion of the German section from the Theosophical Society. February 2–3: Foundation meeting of the Anthroposophical Society. Board members include: Marie von Sivers, Michael Bauer, and Carl Unger. September 20: Laying of the foundation stone for the *Johannes Bau* (Goetheanum) in Dornach. Building begins immediately. The third mystery drama, *The Soul's Awakening* (CW 14), is completed. Also: *The Threshold of the Spiritual World* (CW 147). Lecture cycles include: *The Bhagavad Gita and the Epistles of Paul* and *The Esoteric Meaning of the Bhagavad Gita* (CW 146), which the Russian philosopher Nikolai Berdyaev attends; *The Mysteries of the East and of Christianity* (CW 144); *The Effects of Esoteric Development* (CW 145); and *The Fifth Gospel* (CW 148). In May, Rudolf Steiner is in London and Paris, where anthroposophical work continues.

1914:   Building continues on the *Johannes Bau* (Goetheanum) in Dornach, with artists and coworkers from seventeen nations. The general assembly of the Anthroposophical Society takes place. In May, Rudolf Steiner visits Paris, as well as Chartres Cathedral. June 28: assassination in Sarajevo ('Now the catastrophe has happened!'). August 1: War is declared. Rudolf Steiner returns to Germany from Dornach—he will travel back and forth. He writes the last chapter of *The Riddles of Philosophy*. Lecture cycles include: *Human and Cosmic Thought* (CW 151); *Inner Being of Humanity between Death and a New Birth* (CW 153); *Occult Reading and Occult Hearing* (CW 156). December 24: marriage of Rudolf Steiner and Marie von Sivers.

1915:   Building continues. Life after death becomes a major theme, also art. Writes: *Thoughts during a Time of War* (CW 24). Lectures include: *The Secret of Death* (CW 159); *The Uniting of Humanity through the Christ Impulse* (CW 165).

1916:   Rudolf Steiner begins work with Edith Maryon (1872–1924) on the sculpture 'The Representative of Humanity' ('The Group'—Christ, Lucifer, and Ahriman). He also works with the alchemist Alexander von Bernus on the quarterly *Das Reich*. He writes *The Riddle of Humanity* (CW 20). Lectures include: *Necessity and Freedom in World History and Human Action* (CW 166); *Past and Present in the Human Spirit* (CW 167); *The Karma of Vocation* (CW 172); *The Karma of Untruthfulness* (CW 173).

1917: Russian Revolution. The U.S. enters the war. Building continues. Rudolf Steiner delineates the idea of the 'threefold nature of the human being' (in a public lecture March 15) and the 'threefold nature of the social organism' (hammered out in May–June with the help of Otto von Lerchenfeld and Ludwig Polzer-Hoditz in the form of two documents titled *Memoranda*, which were distributed in high places). August–September: Rudolf Steiner writes *The Riddles of the Soul* (CW 20). Also: commentary on 'The Chemical Wedding of Christian Rosenkreutz' for Alexander Bernus (*Das Reich*). Lectures include: *The Karma of Materialism* (CW 176); *The Spiritual Background of the Outer World: The Fall of the Spirits of Darkness* (CW 177).

1918: March 18: peace treaty of Brest-Litovsk—'Now everything will truly enter chaos! What is needed is cultural renewal.' June: Rudolf Steiner visits Karlstein (Grail) Castle outside Prague. Lecture cycle: *From Symptom to Reality in Modern History* (CW 185). In mid-November, Emil Molt, of the Waldorf-Astoria Cigarette Company, has the idea of founding a school for his workers' children.

1919: Focus on the threefold social organism: tireless travel, countless lectures, meetings, and publications. At the same time, a new public stage of Anthroposophy emerges as cultural renewal begins. The coming years will see initiatives in pedagogy, medicine, pharmacology, and agriculture. January 27: threefold meeting: ' We must first of all, with the money we have, found free schools that can bring people what they need.' February: first public eurythmy performance in Zurich. Also: 'Appeal to the German People' (CW 24), circulated March 6 as a newspaper insert. In April, *Towards Social Renewal* (CW 23) appears— 'perhaps the most widely read of all books on politics appearing since the war.' Rudolf Steiner is asked to undertake the 'direction and leadership' of the school founded by the Waldorf-Astoria Company. Rudolf Steiner begins to talk about the 'renewal' of education. May 30: a building is selected and purchased for the future Waldorf School. August–September, Rudolf Steiner gives a lecture course for Waldorf teachers, *The Foundations of Human Experience (Study of Man)* (CW 293). September 7: Opening of the first Waldorf School. December (into January): first science course, the *Light Course* (CW 320).

1920: The Waldorf School flourishes. New threefold initiatives. Founding of limited companies *Der Kommende Tag* and *Futurum A.G.* to infuse spiritual values into the economic realm. Rudolf Steiner also focuses on the sciences. Lectures: *Introducing Anthroposophical Medicine* (CW 312); *The Warmth Course* (CW 321); *The Boundaries of Natural Science* (CW 322); *The Redemption of Thinking* (CW 74). February: Johannes Werner

Klein—later a cofounder of the Christian Community—asks Rudolf Steiner about the possibility of a 'religious renewal,' a 'Johannine church.' In March, Rudolf Steiner gives the first course for doctors and medical students. In April, a divinity student asks Rudolf Steiner a second time about the possibility of religious renewal. September 27–October 16: anthroposophical 'university course.' December: lectures titled *The Search for the New Isis* (CW 202).

1921:   Rudolf Steiner continues his intensive work on cultural renewal, including the uphill battle for the threefold social order. 'University' arts, scientific, theological, and medical courses include: *The Astronomy Course* (CW 323); *Observation, Mathematics, and Scientific Experiment* (CW 324); the *Second Medical Course* (CW 313); *Color*. In June and September-October, Rudolf Steiner also gives the first two 'priests' courses' (CW 342 and 343). The 'youth movement' gains momentum. Magazines are founded: *Die Drei* (January), and—under the editorship of Albert Steffen (1884–1963)—the weekly, *Das Goetheanum* (August). In February–March, Rudolf Steiner takes his first trip outside Germany since the war (Holland). On April 7, Steiner receives a letter regarding 'religious renewal,' and May 22–23, he agrees to address the question in a practical way. In June, the Klinical-Therapeutic Institute opens in Arlesheim under the direction of Dr. Ita Wegman. In August, the Chemical-Pharmaceutical Laboratory opens in Arlesheim (Oskar Schmiedel and Ita Wegman are directors). The Clinical Therapeutic Institute is inaugurated in Stuttgart (Dr. Ludwig Noll is director); also the Research Laboratory in Dornach (Ehrenfried Pfeiffer and Gunther Wachsmuth are directors). In November–December, Rudolf Steiner visits Norway.

1922:   The first half of the year involves very active public lecturing (thousands attend); in the second half, Rudolf Steiner begins to withdraw and turn toward the Society—'The Society is asleep.' It is 'too weak' to do what is asked of it. The businesses—*Der Kommende Tag* and *Futurum A.G.*—fail. In January, with the help of an agent, Steiner undertakes a twelve-city German lecture tour, accompanied by eurythmy performances. In two weeks he speaks to more than 2,000 people. In April, he gives a 'university course' in The Hague. He also visits England. In June, he is in Vienna for the East–West Congress. In August–September, he is back in England for the Oxford Conference on Education. Returning to Dornach, he gives the lectures *Philosophy, Cosmology, and Religion* (CW 215), and gives the third priests' course (CW 344). On September 16, The Christian Community is founded. In October–November, Steiner is in Holland and England. He also speaks to the youth: *The Youth Course* (CW 217). In December, Steiner gives lectures titled *The Origins of Natural Science* (CW 326), and *Humanity and the World of Stars: The Spiritual Communion of Humanity* (CW 219). December 31: Fire at the Goetheanum, which is destroyed.

1923:   Despite the fire, Rudolf Steiner continues his work unabated. A very hard year. Internal dispersion, dissension, and apathy abound. There is conflict—between old and new visions—within the Society. A wake-up call is needed, and Rudolf Steiner responds with renewed lecturing vitality. His focus: the spiritual context of human life; initiation science; the course of the year; and community building. As a foundation for an artistic school, he creates a series of pastel sketches. Lecture cycles: *The Anthroposophical Movement; Initiation Science* (CW 227) (in England at the Penmaenmawr Summer School); *The Four Seasons and the Archangels* (CW 229); *Harmony of the Creative Word* (CW 230); *The Supersensible Human* (CW 231), given in Holland for the founding of the Dutch society. On November 10, in response to the failed Hitler-Ludendorf putsch in Munich, Steiner closes his Berlin residence and moves the *Philosophisch-Anthroposophisch Verlag* (Press) to Dornach. On December 9, Steiner begins the serialization of his *Autobiography: The Course of My Life* (CW 28) in *Das Goetheanum*. It will continue to appear weekly, without a break, until his death. Late December–early January: Rudolf Steiner re-founds the Anthroposophical Society (about 12,000 members internationally) and takes over its leadership. The new board members are: Marie Steiner, Ita Wegman, Albert Steffen, Elizabeth Vreede, and Guenther Wachsmuth. (See *The Christmas Meeting for the Founding of the General Anthroposophical Society*, CW 260). Accompanying lectures: *Mystery Knowledge and Mystery Centers* (CW 232); *World History in the Light of Anthroposophy* (CW 233). December 25: the Foundation Stone is laid (in the hearts of members) in the form of the 'Foundation Stone Meditation.'

1924: January 1: having founded the Anthroposophical Society and taken over its leadership, Rudolf Steiner has the task of 'reforming' it. The process begins with a weekly newssheet ('What's Happening in the Anthroposophical Society') in which Rudolf Steiner's 'Letters to Members' and 'Anthroposophical Leading Thoughts' appear (CW 26). The next step is the creation of a new esoteric class, the 'first class' of the 'University of Spiritual Science' (which was to have been followed, had Rudolf Steiner lived longer, by two more advanced classes). Then comes a new language for Anthroposophy—practical, phenomenological, and direct; and Rudolf Steiner creates the model for the second Goetheanum. He begins the series of extensive 'karma' lectures (CW 235–40); and finally, responding to needs, he creates two new initiatives: biodynamic agriculture and curative education. After the middle of the year, rumors begin to circulate regarding Steiner's health. Lectures: January–February, *Anthroposophy* (CW 234); February: *Tone Eurythmy* (CW 278); June: *The Agriculture Course* (CW 327); June–July: *Speech Eurythmy* (CW 279); *Curative Education* (CW 317); August: (England, 'Second International Summer School'), *Initiation Consciousness: True and False Paths in Spiritual Investigation* (CW 243); September: *Pastoral Medicine* (CW 318). On September 26, for the first time, Rudolf Steiner cancels a lecture. On September 28, he gives his last lecture. On September 29, he withdraws to his studio in the carpenter's shop; now he is definitively ill. Cared for by Ita Wegman, he continues working, however, and writing the weekly installments of his *Autobiography* and *Letters to the Members/Leading Thoughts* (CW 26).

1925: Rudolf Steiner, while continuing to work, continues to weaken. He finishes *Extending Practical Medicine* (CW 27) with Ita Wegman.
On March 30, around ten in the morning, Rudolf Steiner dies.

INDEX

PLATES

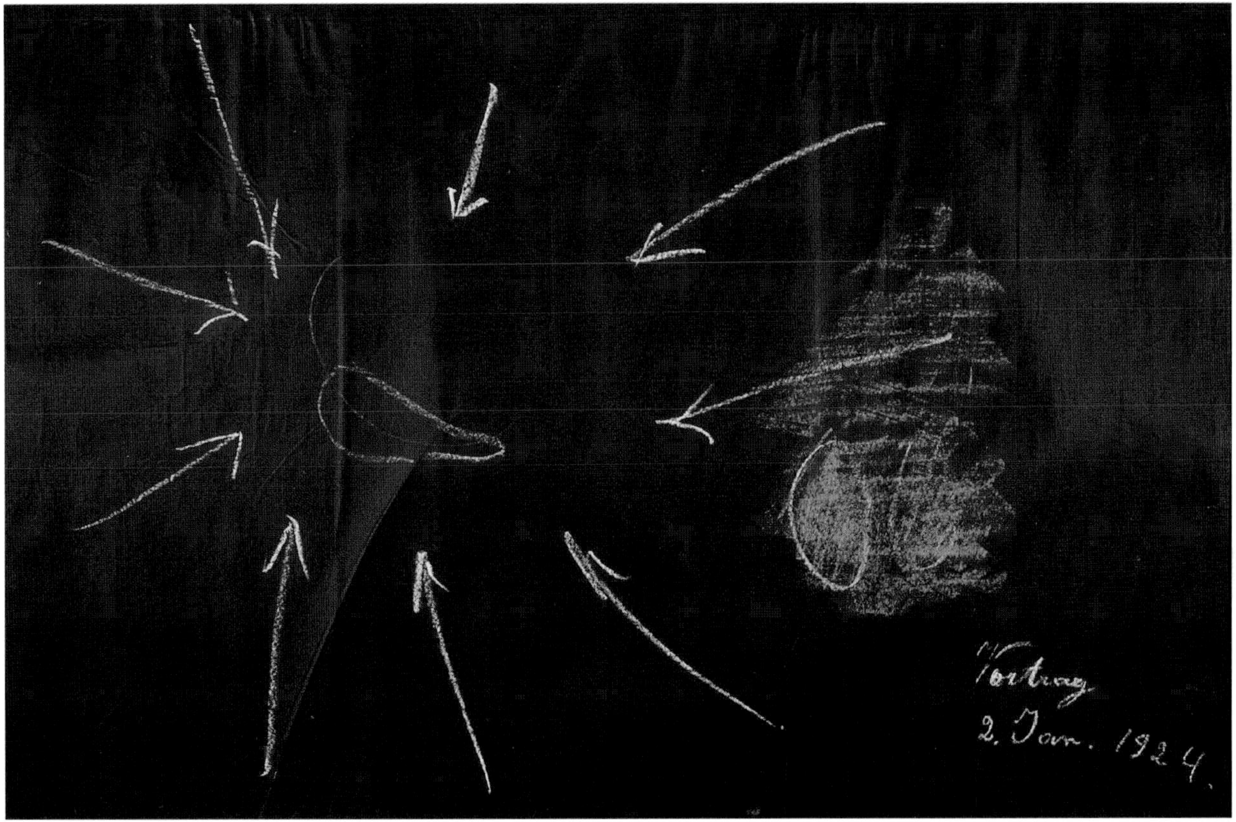

Plate 1

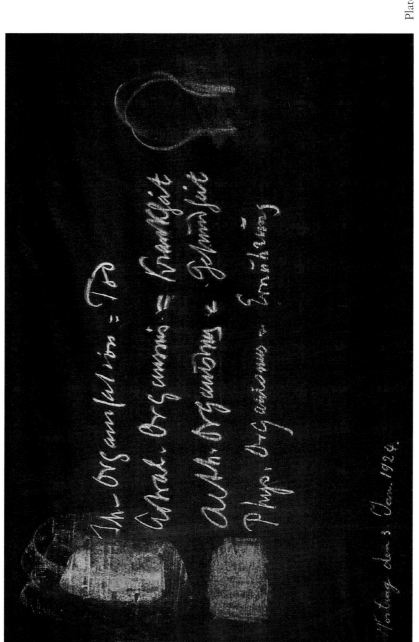

Plate 2

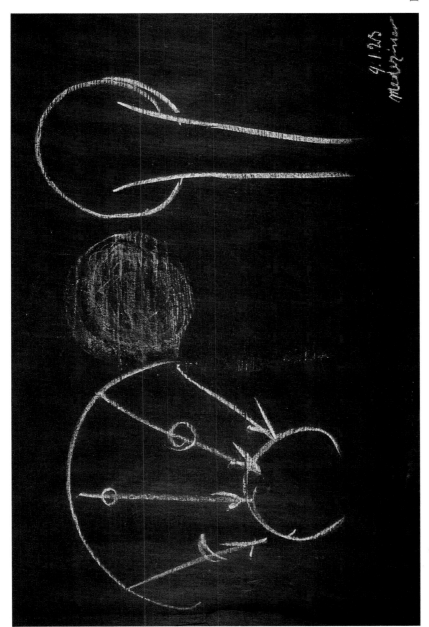

Plate 3

Plate 4

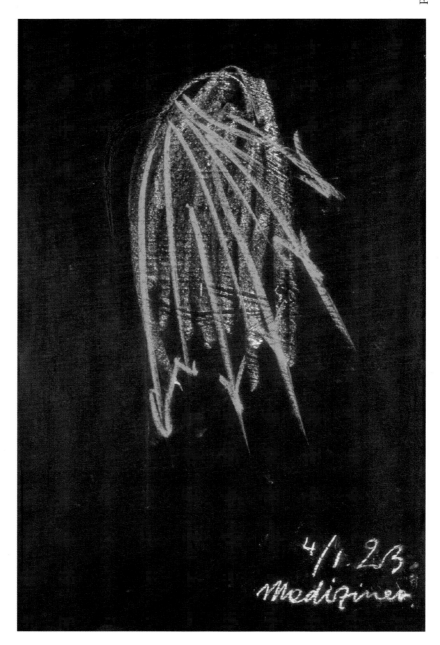

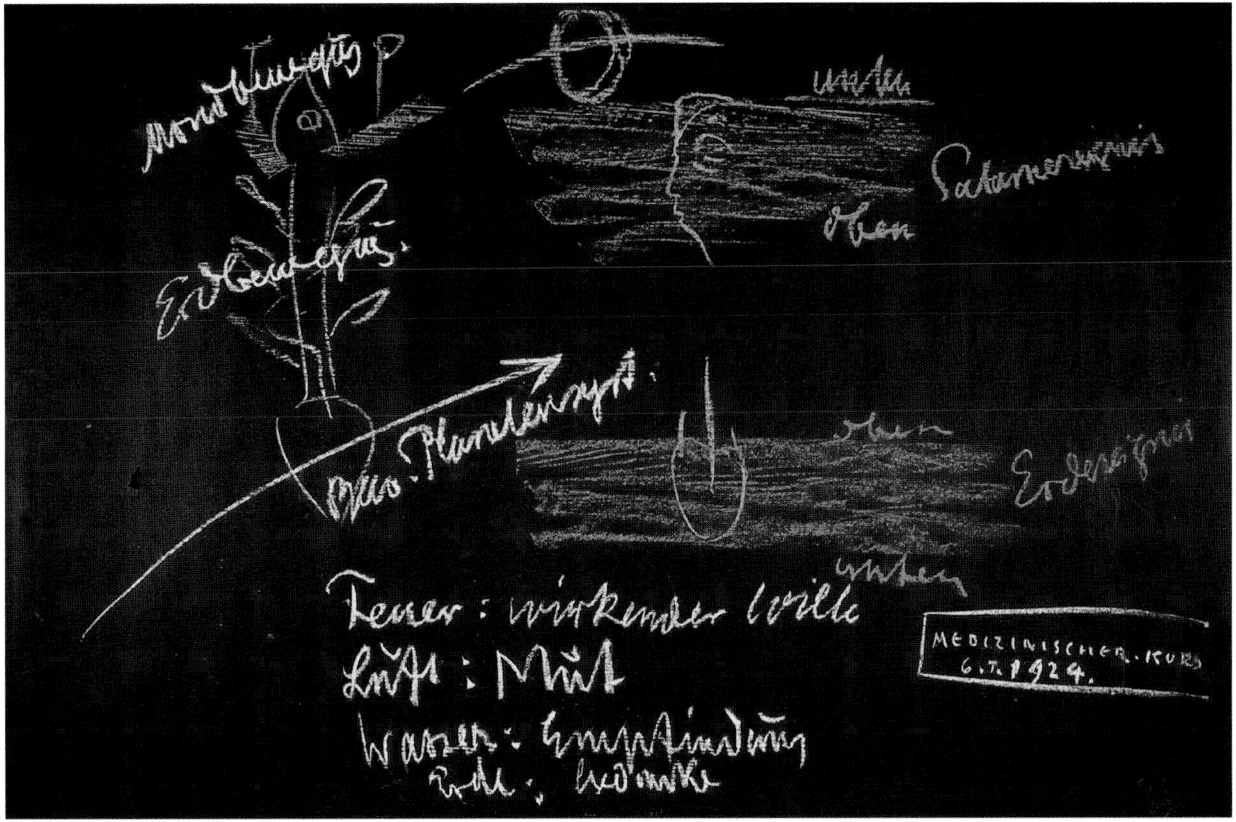
unten
oben
oben
unten
Feuer : wirkender Wille
Luft : Mut
Wasser : Empfindung
Erde : Gedanke
MEDIZINISCHER KURS
6.IV.1924.

Plate 5

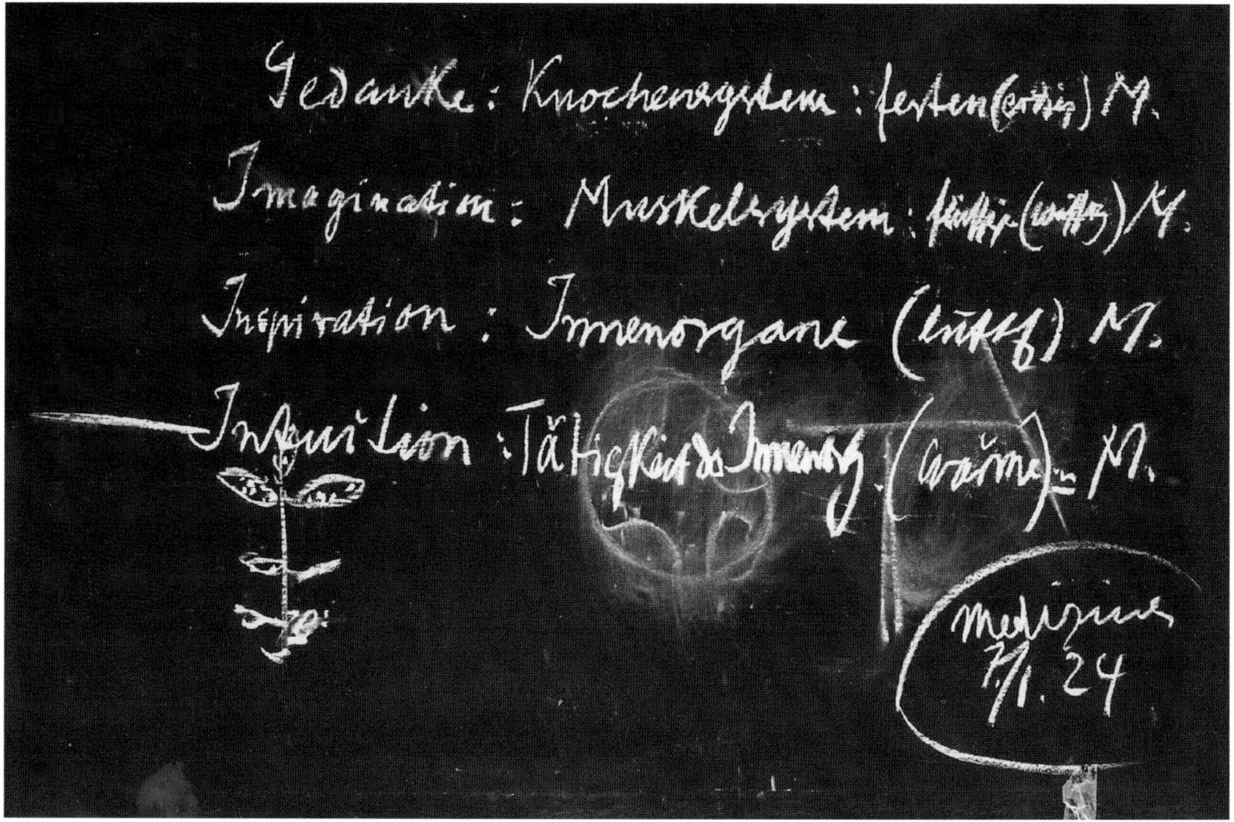
Gedanke : Knochensystem : festen
Imagination : Muskelsystem
Inspiration : Innenorgane
Intuition : Tätigkeit d. Innenorg.
(wärme)
7/1. 24

Plate 6

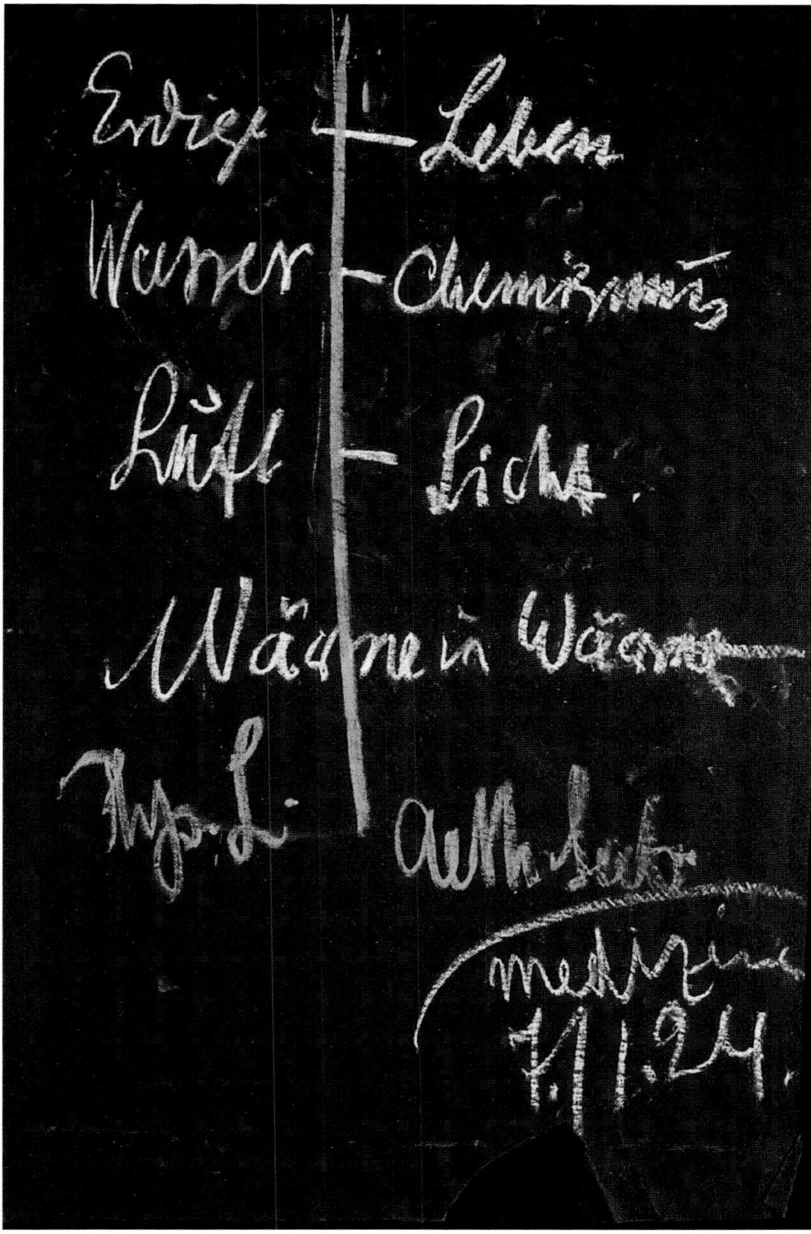

Plate 7

Plate 8

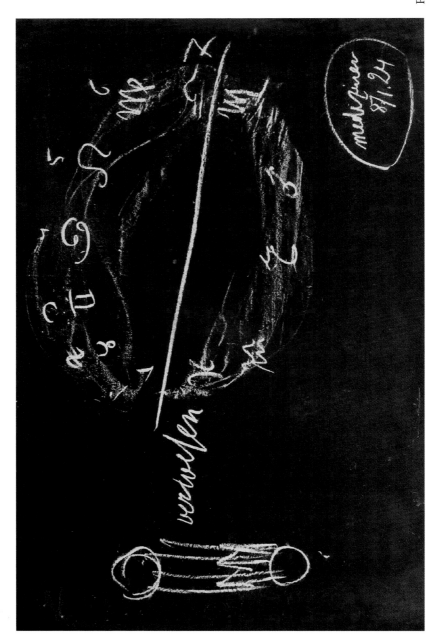

Plate 9

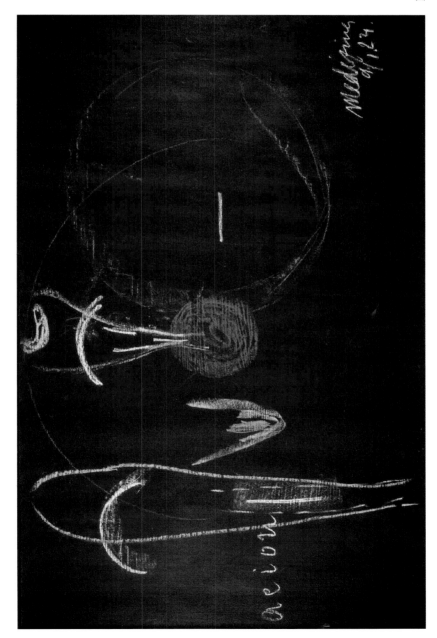

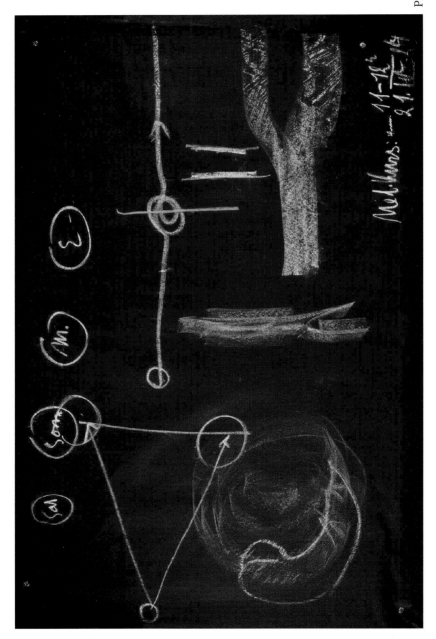

Plate 10

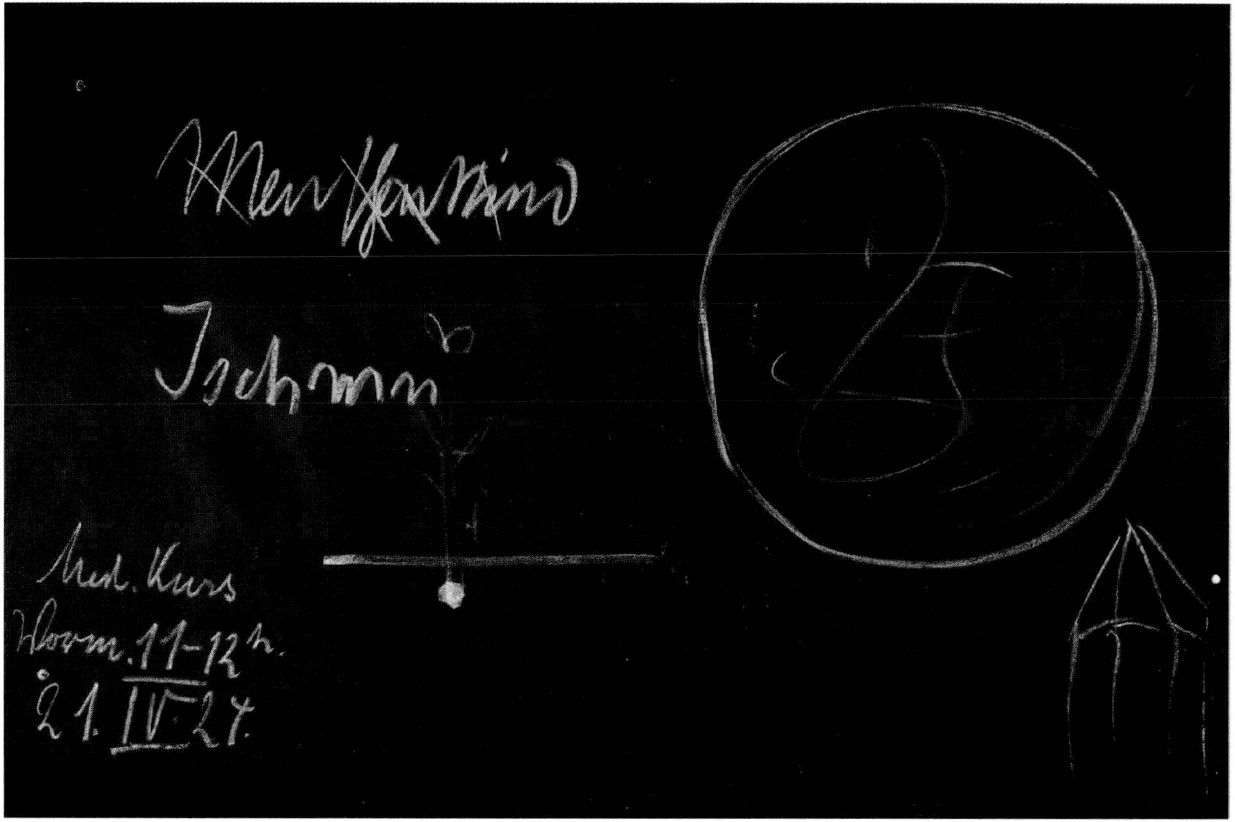

Plate 11

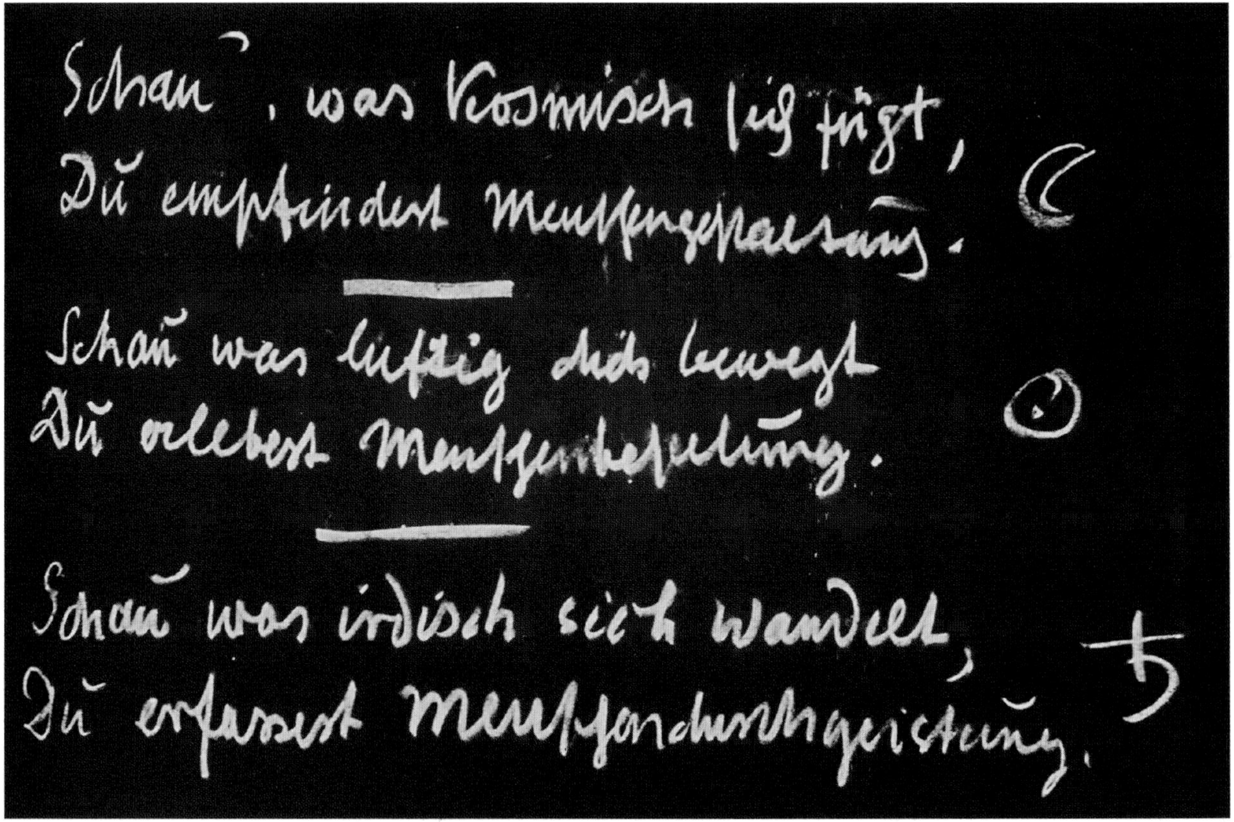
Schau, was kosmisch sich fügt,
Du empfindest Menschengestaltung.
Schau was luftig dich bewegt
Du erlebest Menschenbeseelung.
Schau was irdisch sich wandelt,
Du erfassest Menschendurchgeistung.

Plate 12

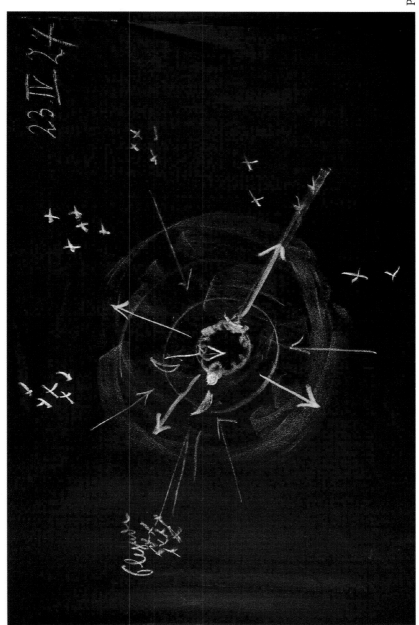

Plate 13

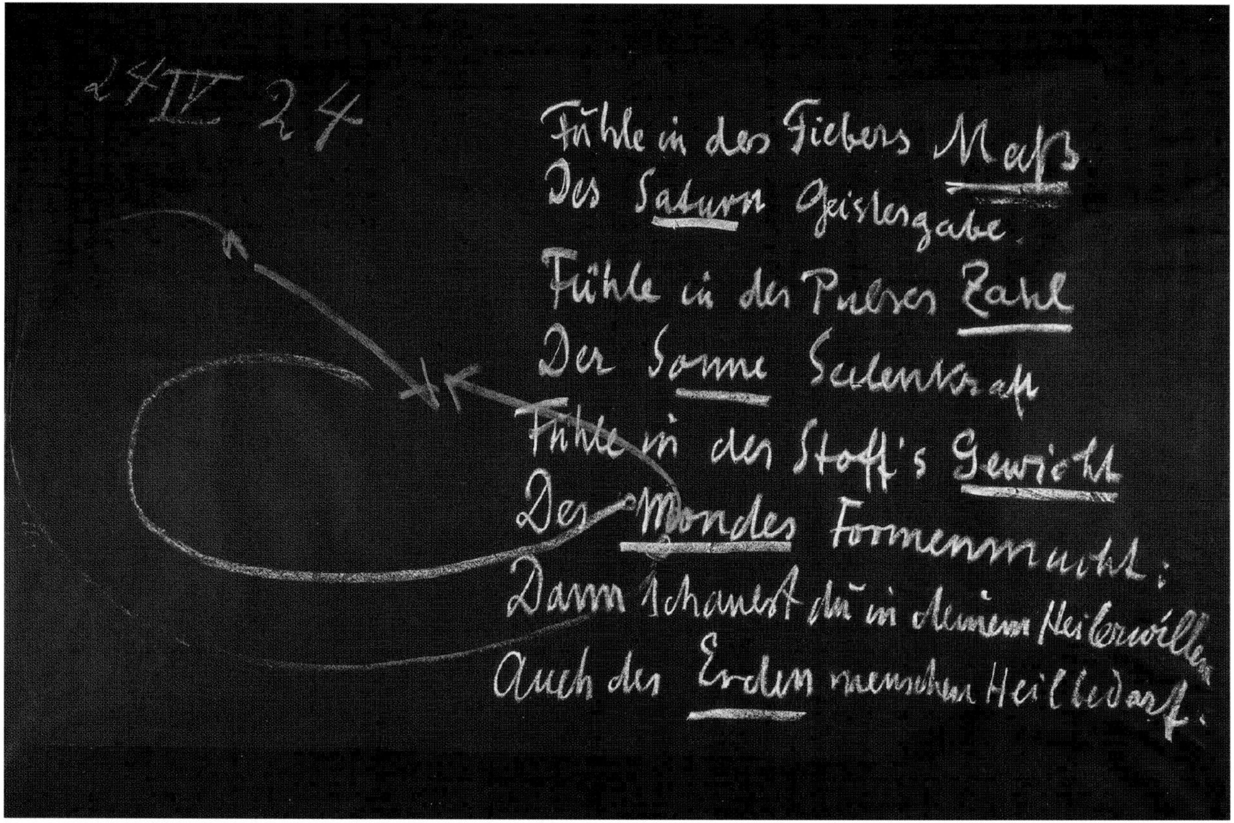

Plate 14

24 IV 24

Fühle in des Fiebers Maß
Des Saturn Geistesgabe.

Fühle in der Pulsen Rad
Der Sonne Seelenkraft

Fühle in ein Stoff's Gewicht
Des Mondes Formenmacht;

Dann schaust du in deinem Heilewillen
Auch den Erdenmenschen Heilbedarf.

Plate 15

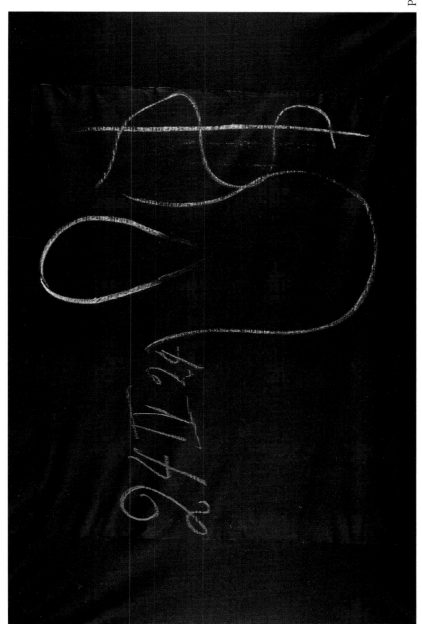

Schaue die Frühzeit
In der Kinder Leben,
Und der Kinder erste
In die Jugendzeit:
Dir erscheint verdichtet
Menschenætherisein
Hinter Körperwesen

Schaue die Lebensschicht
In die Menschen reifezeit,
Und an Reife alter
In den Jugendleben;
Dir wird in Wellenklängen
Menschenseelenwirken
Aus dem ætherleben;

25 IV 24

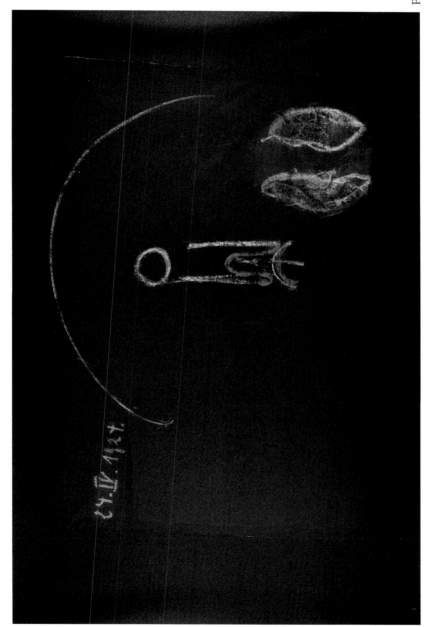

Plate 18

Plate 19

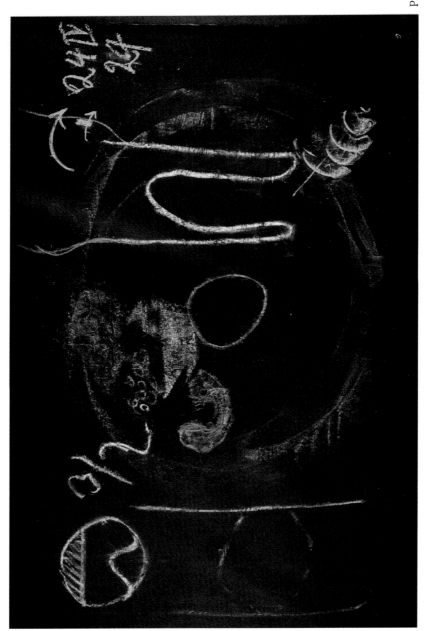